AI in Healthcare:

Empowering Doctors and Administrators

Abdul Gafur Mundoli

notionpress.com

INDIA • SINGAPORE • MALAYSIA

ISBN

Hardcase 979-8-89724-866-7
Paperback 979-8-89724-865-0

CONTENTS

PREFACE

In the rapidly evolving landscape of healthcare, few innovations hold as much promise as artificial intelligence. "AI in Healthcare: Empowering Doctors and Administrators" is a comprehensive guide tailored specifically for dedicated professionals at the heart of healthcare delivery—doctors, nurses, students, healthcare administrators, entrepreneurs and policymakers. This book offers them a detailed exploration of how AI can be effectively implemented to enhance patient care and improve operational efficiencies.

As AI continues to evolve, its capabilities in diagnosing diseases, personalizing treatment plans, predicting patient outcomes, and streamlining administrative processes become increasingly vital. This book aims to demystify AI, providing a clear roadmap for its integration into everyday medical practice and healthcare management.

We begin with an overview of AI fundamentals, ensuring that readers have a solid grasp of key concepts and terminologies and explore different stages of AI workflow, from data collection to deployment. Understanding this workflow is crucial for effectively integrating AI into healthcare settings.

In this book we examine how AI addresses current challenges in the healthcare system, such as limited doctor-patient interaction, outdated practices, healthcare costs, and data overload. By showcasing tangible examples, we aim to inspire and guide healthcare professionals in envisioning how they can apply similar technologies within their own practices.

In addition to practical applications, we address the critical ethical and regulatory considerations surrounding AI in healthcare. Issues such as patient privacy, data security, and algorithmic bias are discussed comprehensively, providing a balanced view of the challenges and responsibilities that come with AI integration.

It is my sincere hope that this book will serve as a valuable resource, inspiring you to explore the possibilities of AI and ultimately, to improve the health and well-being of patients everywhere.

Thank you for embarking on this journey with me. Together, let us explore the transformative potential of AI in healthcare and work towards a future of smarter, more efficient, and compassionate medical care.

– Dr Abdul Gafur Mundoli

Chapter 01

FOUNDATIONS OF AI

In today's rapidly evolving healthcare landscape, a profound understanding of fundamental artificial intelligence concepts is essential. AI is fundamentally changing how healthcare is delivered, diagnosed, and treated. This chapter aims to equip healthcare professionals, administrators, and aspiring entrepreneurs with essential knowledge to comprehend the intricacies of AI. Topics covered include the basics of AI, the fundamentals of machine learning and deep learning, as well as an overview of natural language processing (NLP) and computer vision. This knowledge is crucial for healthcare practitioners, administrators, and entrepreneurs in the healthcare industry.

1.1 Basics of Artificial Intelligence

1.1.1 Defining Artificial Intelligence

Artificial Intelligence is the branch of computer science dedicated to creating systems and machines capable of performing tasks that typically require human intelligence. These tasks may include learning from experience, reasoning based on that knowledge, solving complex problems, understanding natural language, and perceiving and interacting with the environment. AI systems are designed to mimic human cognitive functions, enabling them to adapt and evolve in response to new data, make predictions, recognize patterns, and perform tasks traditionally requiring human intelligence.

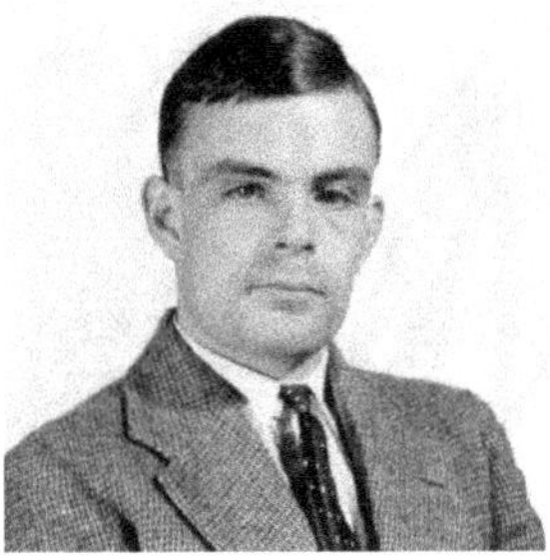

Alan Turing

Alan Turing, a British mathematician, logician, and computer scientist, was instrumental in the development and conceptualization of Artificial Intelligence. In 1950, Turing introduced the renowned Turing Test as a criterion for determining whether a machine exhibits human-like intelligence. According to the test, if a human evaluator interacting with a computer via a text-based interface cannot distinguish whether they are communicating with a human or a machine, then the machine can be deemed to exhibit intelligence.

Turing's contributions were foundational to the field of AI, as he approached the concept of intelligence by focusing on observable actions rather than abstract definitions. His ideas also stimulated research in crucial AI areas like natural language processing and machine learning, which are fundamental components of today's AI systems. Moreover, Turing's impact on computer science extended through his invention of the Turing machine, which established the theoretical framework for modern computing and influenced the early design of AI systems.

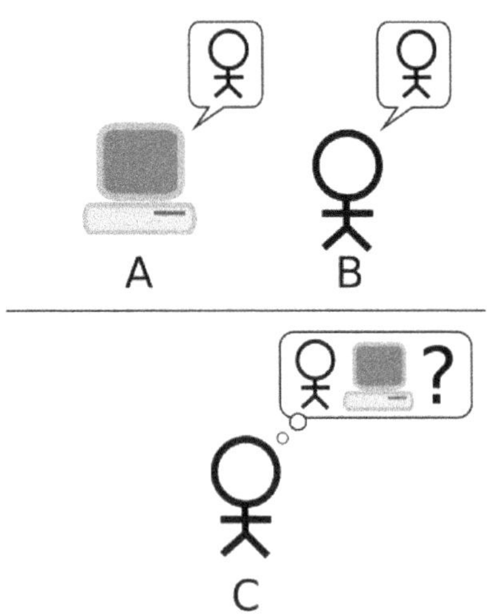

Turing Test

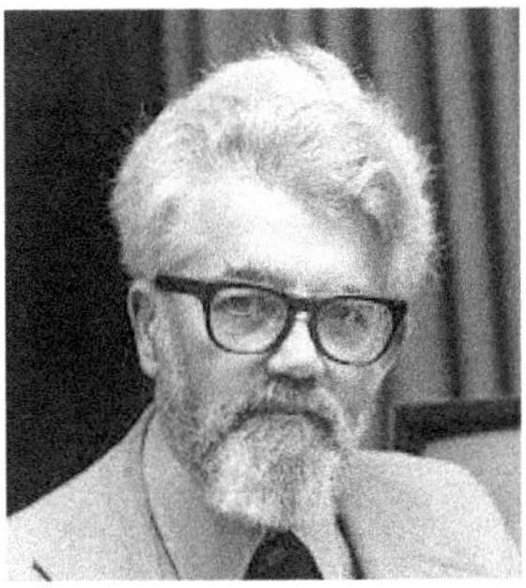

John McCarthy

The term "Artificial Intelligence" was coined by John McCarthy in 1956 at the Dartmouth Conference, where he and other pioneers in the field explored the potential of developing machines capable of simulating human intelligence. McCarthy defined AI as "the science and engineering of making intelligent machines." Since then, AI has evolved significantly, with milestones including the development of expert systems in the 1970s, the emergence of neural networks and machine learning in the 1980s and 1990s, and the recent advancements in deep learning and reinforcement learning techniques. Today, AI permeates virtually every aspect of modern life, from virtual assistants like Siri and Alexa to self-driving cars, and extends into finance, e-commerce, healthcare, education, manufacturing, transportation, logistics, and customer service, demonstrating its profound impact on society and technology.

1.1.2 Uses of Artificial Intelligence

Artificial Intelligence has rapidly evolved from a futuristic idea into a practical and integral part of our daily lives, revolutionizing various industries and sectors. Here are some significant uses of AI across different domains:

1. Healthcare

The emergence of artificial intelligence in healthcare has been groundbreaking, reshaping the way we diagnose, treat and monitor patients. This technology is drastically improving healthcare research and outcomes by producing more accurate diagnoses and enabling more personalized treatments. AI in healthcare's ability to analyse vast amounts of clinical documentation quickly helps medical professionals identify disease markers and trends that might otherwise go unnoticed. For healthcare facility owners, AI offers substantial benefits as well. It can optimize operational efficiency by streamlining administrative tasks such as scheduling, resource allocation, and inventory management. AI-driven analytics can also help in predicting patient flow and optimizing staffing levels, ensuring that resources are allocated efficiently and patient care is optimized. The potential applications of AI and healthcare are broad and far-reaching, from scanning radiological images for early detection to predicting outcomes from electronic health records. Listed below are a few of many applications.

- Medical Diagnosis: AI algorithms analyse various types of medical data, such as symptoms, medical imaging, and patient history, to support healthcare professionals in diagnosing diseases more accurately and quickly. For instance, AI-powered diagnostic tools can analyse X-rays, MRIs, and CT scans to identify abnormalities.
- Drug Discovery: AI speeds up the drug discovery process by analysing huge datasets to identify potential drug candidates, predict their efficacy, and optimize their properties. This helps in cutting down the time and cost involved in bringing new drugs to market.
- Predictive Analysis of Diseases: AI models can analyse patient data to predict the probability of developing certain diseases or medical conditions. This enables proactive interventions and personalized healthcare plans to mitigate risks.
- Personalized Treatment Recommendations: AI-powered systems can analyse individual patient data, including genetic information, medical history, and treatment outcomes, to recommend customised treatment plans designed for each patient's specific needs and characteristics.
- Patient Monitoring: AI-powered monitoring systems continuously analyse patient data, such as vital signs, lab results, and medication adherence, to detect early warning signs of deterioration or complications, enabling timely interventions.

- Optimizing Operational Workflows: AI algorithms optimize hospital operations by streamlining administrative tasks, managing appointment schedules, allocating resources efficiently, and predicting patient admissions and discharge patterns. These enhancements boost overall efficiency and cut down on expenses.
- Improving Healthcare Outcomes: By leveraging AI for data-driven decision-making, healthcare providers can improve patient outcomes, reduce medical errors, and enhance the quality and efficiency of healthcare delivery.

2. Finance

Artificial Intelligence is rapidly transforming the finance industry, revolutionizing the way financial institutions operate and profoundly impacting various aspects of finance. The integration of AI in finance has brought forth numerous benefits of AI in finance, and nowadays, there is a broad spectrum of AI applications in finance that can prove to be game changers in the future of finance industry. Listed below are a few of many applications.

- Credit Scoring: AI algorithms analyse huge amounts of financial data to assess the creditworthiness of individuals and businesses. By considering various factors such as credit history, income, debt-to-income ratio, and spending patterns, AI systems can accurately predict the risk of default and assign appropriate credit scores.
- Fraud Detection: AI-powered fraud detection systems analyse transaction data in real-time to identify suspicious patterns and anomalies indicative of fraudulent activities, such as unauthorized transactions, identity theft, or money laundering. By detecting and preventing fraud early, financial institutions can minimize financial losses and protect their customers.
- Financial Forecasting: AI models analyse historical financial data, market trends, economic indicators, and other relevant factors to generate forecasts and predictions regarding asset prices,

stock market movements, currency fluctuations, and economic conditions. These forecasts assist investors, traders, and financial institutions in making informed decisions and managing risks effectively.

3. Retail

AI is revolutionizing retail by enabling personalized customer experiences, optimizing operational efficiency, and predicting market trends with unprecedented accuracy. These advancements are reshaping how retailers engage with consumers and adapt to evolving market dynamics, fostering a more agile and competitive industry landscape. Listed below are a few of many applications.

- Product Recommendations: AI-powered recommendation systems analyse customer data, such as purchase history, browsing behaviour, and demographic information, to suggest products that are likely to be of interest to individual shoppers. These recommendations can be provided through online platforms, personalized emails, or targeted advertisements, enhancing the shopping experience and increasing sales.
- Price Optimization: AI algorithms analyse various factors, including demand patterns, competitor pricing, inventory levels, and historical sales data, to dynamically adjust prices in real-time. This enables retailers to optimize pricing strategies, maximize revenue, and maintain competitiveness in the market.
- Supply Chain Management: AI is utilized in supply chain management to improve inventory management, demand forecasting, and logistics optimization. AI algorithms analyse data from suppliers, distributors, and retailers to predict demand fluctuations, optimize inventory levels, and streamline logistics operations, reducing costs and improving efficiency throughout the supply chain.

4. Manufacturing

Artificial intelligence is changing the manufacturing industry lock, stock, and barrel with its transformative capabilities. Major manufacturing businesses are leveraging the power of AI to increase efficiency, accuracy, and productivity across various processes. Listed below are a few of many applications.

- Quality Control: AI-powered systems inspect products during the manufacturing process using AI techniques such as computer vision and sensor data analysis. These systems detect defects, deviations from specifications, and other quality issues in real-time, allowing manufacturers to take corrective actions promptly and ensure that only high-quality products reach the market.
- Predictive Maintenance: AI algorithms analyse sensor data, equipment performance metrics, and historical maintenance records to predict equipment failures and maintenance needs before they occur. By identifying potential issues in advance, manufacturers can schedule maintenance activities more efficiently, minimize unplanned downtime, and extend the lifespan of machinery and equipment.
- Production Optimization: AI is used to optimize various aspects of the production process, such as scheduling, resource allocation, and workflow management. AI-driven optimization algorithms consider factors such as production goals, resource constraints, and market demand to maximize production efficiency, minimize costs, and improve overall productivity.

5. Transportation

Today, the transportation industry has reached an unprecedented level where vehicles don't even require human intervention to zoom around on the road. Obviously, technological advancements have laid a hand in its remarkable journey of innovation and evolution. We are now at the age where AI in transportation helps achieve major breakthroughs, catching the eyes of transportation bosses worldwide. Listed below are a few of many applications.

- Autonomous Vehicles: AI plays a crucial role in the development and operation of autonomous vehicles (AVs). AVs utilize various AI technologies, including computer vision, machine learning, and sensor fusion, to perceive their surroundings, interpret traffic signals, and make driving decisions in real-time. AI algorithms enable AVs to navigate safely, avoid obstacles, and adapt to changing road conditions, ultimately leading to safer and more efficient transportation systems.
- Traffic Prediction: AI models analyse historical traffic data, weather conditions, events, and other relevant factors to predict traffic patterns and congestion levels in different areas. These predictions help transportation authorities and commuters plan routes, avoid traffic jams, and reduce travel time.
- Route Optimization: AI-powered route optimization algorithms consider factors such as traffic conditions, road closures, vehicle capacities, and delivery schedules to find the most efficient routes for transportation fleets, including trucks, delivery vehicles, and ride-sharing services. By optimizing routes, AI helps reduce fuel consumption, minimize vehicle idle time, and improve overall fleet efficiency.

6. Customer Service

Ensuring customer engagement and retention is a key concern for businesses in theBusiness-to-Consumer (B2C) sector, especially as digital platforms disrupt traditional models. Engaged customers exhibit higher loyalty, interact more frequently with brands, and ultimately contribute greater lifetime value. AI-powered customer service has emerged as the most efficient method for organizations to provide tailored, proactive experiences that enhance customer engagement. Below are a few examples of its many uses.

- AI-Powered Chatbots: AI-powered chatbots are virtual assistants that use natural language processing (NLP) and machine learning algorithms to interact with customers in real-time. Chatbots can answer frequently asked questions, provide product recommendations, assist with order tracking, and handle routine inquiries, freeing up human agents to focus on more complex issues. By offering instant support and round-the-clock availability, AI-powered chatbots enhance the customer service experience and increase customer satisfaction.
- Handling Simple Requests: Chatbots are particularly effective at handling simple and repetitive customer service tasks, such as account inquiries, password resets, and basic troubleshooting. By automating these tasks, chatbots improve response times, reduce customer wait times, and enhance operational efficiency for businesses.
- Personalized Assistance: AI-powered chatbots can analyse customer interactions and preferences to offer personalized assistance and recommendations. By understanding customer needs and preferences based on past interactions and purchase history, chatbots can provide tailored recommendations, promotions, and offers, enhancing the overall customer experience and driving sales.

7. Security

AI security solutions have become robust tools for detecting and countering potential threats in the current digital environment. Using machine learning and deep learning algorithms, AI can scrutinize large datasets, identify suspicious activities, and offer organizations heightened defenses against cyber attacks. Below are few examples of its diverse applications.

- Facial Recognition: AI-powered facial recognition systems analyse facial features from images or video footage to identify individuals. These systems are used for various security applications, including access control, surveillance, and identity verification. Facial recognition technology enables secure authentication and monitoring in areas such as airports, government facilities, and commercial buildings.

- Intrusion Detection: AI algorithms analyse network traffic patterns, system logs, and user behaviour to detect suspicious activities indicative of unauthorized access or cyber threats. Intrusion detection systems (IDS) and intrusion prevention systems (IPS) leverage AI techniques, such as anomaly detection and machine learning, to identify and respond to potential security breaches in real-time, protecting networks and data assets from cyber attacks.
- Cyber Security Threat Analysis: AI-powered threat intelligence platforms analyse vast amounts of data from diverse sources, including malware samples, network traffic, and security logs, to identify emerging cyber threats and vulnerabilities. These platforms use machine learning and data analytics to correlate and analyse security events, prioritize alerts, and provide actionable insights to security analysts, enabling proactive threat mitigation and incident response.

8. Marketing

AI is a powerful tool for marketers. Using AI for marketing allows you to gain insights into customer behavior and customize the timing, targeting, and content of marketing efforts. Below are some examples among numerous applications. Listed below are a few of many applications.

- Targeted Advertising: AI algorithms analyse consumer data, such as demographics, browsing history, and purchase behaviour, to deliver personalized advertisements tailored to individual preferences and interests. By targeting relevant audiences with customized ads, marketers can improve ad engagement, conversion rates, and return on investment (ROI).

- Customer Segmentation: AI-driven segmentation techniques categorize customers into distinct groups based on shared characteristics, such as demographics, behaviour, and preferences. By segmenting the target audience effectively, marketers can tailor marketing campaigns, messages, and offers to each segment's specific needs and interests, improving campaign effectiveness and customer engagement.
- Sentiment Analysis: AI-powered sentiment analysis tools analyse text data from social media, customer reviews, and other sources to understand the sentiment, opinions, and emotions expressed by customers about products, brands, or topics. By monitoring sentiment trends and identifying positive or negative feedback, marketers can gauge customer satisfaction, identify areas for improvement, and adjust marketing strategies accordingly to better meet customer expectations.

9. Education

Artificial Intelligence has the capability to fundamentally transform the landscape of education and how teaching and learning are conducted. By using AI-powered tools and strategies, educators can personalize learning, improve student outcomes, and better prepare students for success in the digital age. Here are a few examples among its many applications.

- Personalized Learning: AI-powered educational platforms utilize machine learning algorithms to adapt learning materials and experiences to the individual needs, preferences, and learning styles of each student. By analysing student performance data, such as assessment results, engagement patterns, and learning progress, AI algorithms can recommend personalized learning pathways, resources, and activities tailored to each student's strengths, weaknesses, and interests. Personalized learning promotes self-paced learning, enhances student engagement, and improves learning outcomes by providing targeted support and scaffolding to address individual learning needs.

- Adaptive Testing: AI-driven adaptive testing platforms use machine learning algorithms to dynamically adjust the difficulty and content of assessments based on the performance of individual test-takers. Adaptive tests present questions tailored to the test-taker's skill level and performance, gradually increasing or decreasing the difficulty level based on their responses. By adapting the test content in real-time, adaptive testing maximizes the precision and efficiency of assessment, accurately measuring students' knowledge, skills, and competencies while minimizing test-taking time and reducing test anxiety.
- Intelligent Tutoring Systems: AI-powered intelligent tutoring systems (ITS) provide personalized, interactive learning experiences that emulate one-on-one tutoring interactions between students and human tutors. ITS leverage natural language processing (NLP), machine learning, and cognitive modelling techniques to assess student understanding, provide real-time feedback, and deliver customized instruction and support. By adapting instructional strategies, pacing, and content delivery to individual student needs, ITS enhance learning effectiveness, promote mastery learning, and facilitate deeper conceptual understanding across various subjects and domains.

1.1.3 Drawbacks of Artificial Intelligence

While AI has made significant strides in reshaping paradigms and augmenting capabilities, it is not without its drawbacks. Understanding the limitations and potential pitfalls of AI is crucial for navigating its integration into our daily lives and societal frameworks. Listed below are a few of its limitations.

a) Bias and unfairness: Bias and unfairness are significant concerns in the development and deployment of AI systems. When training data contains biases, whether they are related to race, gender, or other factors, AI systems can inadvertently learn and perpetuate these biases in their decision-making processes. This can lead to discriminatory outcomes, where certain groups are unfairly treated or marginalized by AI-driven decisions. Moreover, the complexity of AI algorithms can make it challenging to identify and address biases effectively. As a result, it is crucial for developers and stakeholders to carefully consider bias mitigation strategies throughout the entire AI lifecycle, from data collection and preprocessing to algorithm design and evaluation. Failure to address bias and unfairness in AI systems can not only undermine trust in these technologies but also have real-world consequences, exacerbating social inequalities and perpetuating systemic discrimination. Therefore, ongoing research and efforts to develop more transparent, accountable, and fair AI systems are essential to ensure that these technologies benefit society as a whole.

Example in Healthcare Context: In the medical context, bias and unfairness in AI systems can have serious implications for patient care. For instance, imagine an AI system designed to assist doctors in diagnosing diseases based on medical imaging scans. If the training data used to develop this AI system primarily consists of scans from a particular demographic group, such as individuals of a certain ethnicity or gender, the system may inadvertently learn biases present in those datasets.

As a result, when the AI system is deployed in real-world clinical settings, it may be more accurate in diagnosing conditions in patients who match the demographic makeup of the training data, while potentially being less accurate for patients from underrepresented groups. This can lead to disparities in healthcare outcomes, with certain patients receiving delayed or incorrect diagnoses due to the biases embedded in the AI system.

Moreover, biases in AI systems can also affect treatment recommendations. For example, if historical data used to train an AI-driven treatment recommendation system reflects disparities in the treatment provided to different demographic groups, the system may inadvertently propagate those disparities by recommending treatments that favour certain groups over others.

Addressing bias and unfairness in medical AI systems is critical to ensure equitable access to healthcare and to mitigate the risk of exacerbating existing healthcare disparities. This may involve diversifying training data to better represent the patient population, implementing bias detection and mitigation techniques during the development of AI algorithms, and continually evaluating and refining these systems to minimize the impact of bias on patient care.

b) The lack of transparency and accountability in complex AI systems poses significant challenges in various domains, including finance, criminal justice, and healthcare. Without clear insight into the inner workings of AI algorithms, it becomes difficult for stakeholders, including policymakers, regulators, and end-users, to understand how decisions are being made and to assess the fairness and reliability of those decisions.

This opacity can lead to concerns about algorithmic bias, where discriminatory outcomes may occur without clear visibility into the factors influencing decision-making. Additionally, the lack of transparency can hinder efforts to identify and rectify errors or biases in AI systems, potentially resulting in unjust or harmful consequences for individuals affected by these systems.

Furthermore, the absence of accountability mechanisms can exacerbate these issues, as there may be no clear recourse for individuals who are adversely impacted by AI-driven decisions. This can erode trust in AI technologies and lead to resistance or scepticism towards their adoption and deployment in critical applications.

Addressing the lack of transparency and accountability in AI systems requires concerted efforts from developers, researchers, policymakers, and other stakeholders. This may involve initiatives to enhance the interpretability of AI algorithms, such as developing explainable AI techniques that provide insights into the decision-making process. Additionally, establishing robust mechanisms for auditing and oversight can help ensure that AI systems are held accountable for their actions and that appropriate remedies are available in cases of errors or biases. By promoting greater transparency and accountability in AI development and deployment, we can foster trust and confidence in these technologies while mitigating the risks of unintended consequences.

Example in Healthcare Context: In the medical context, the lack of transparency and accountability in AI systems can be exemplified by the use of black-box algorithms for patient diagnosis or treatment recommendations. For instance, imagine a hospital implementing an AI system to assist radiologists in interpreting medical imaging scans, such as X-rays or MRIs, to detect abnormalities or diseases.

If the AI system utilizes a complex deep learning model or other sophisticated algorithm, it may produce accurate predictions, but without providing clear explanations for how it arrived at those conclusions. In other words, the decision-making process of the AI system is opaque or "black-boxed" to the end-users, including the healthcare providers relying on its recommendations.

In such a scenario, radiologists and other medical professionals may find it challenging to understand why the AI system recommended a particular diagnosis or course of action. They may be unable to ascertain which features or patterns in the imaging data influenced the AI's decision, making it difficult to validate or trust its recommendations fully.

This lack of transparency can have several implications for patient care. Firstly, it may hinder clinicians' ability to critically evaluate the AI system's outputs and potentially lead to scepticism or reluctance to rely on its recommendations. Secondly, it can make it challenging to identify errors or biases in the AI's decision-making process, raising concerns about patient safety and quality of care.

Furthermore, the absence of clear accountability mechanisms means that if the AI system makes a mistake or produces a biased recommendation, it may be difficult to attribute responsibility or take corrective actions.

Addressing these challenges requires the development of explainable AI techniques tailored to the medical domain, allowing clinicians to understand and interpret the reasoning behind AI-driven diagnoses or treatment recommendations. Additionally, establishing robust processes for auditing and validating AI systems can help ensure accountability and mitigate the risks associated with opaque decision-making processes in healthcare. By promoting transparency and accountability in medical AI systems, we can enhance trust, facilitate collaboration between humans and AI, and ultimately improve patient outcomes.

c) Job displacement is a pressing concern stemming from the rapid advancement of AI technology. As AI becomes more sophisticated, it has the capability to automate tasks across various industries, including healthcare, manufacturing, transportation, customer service, and administrative work. This automation can lead to significant job loss, particularly for tasks that are repetitive, routine, and easily codifiable.

Furthermore, the displacement of human workers by AI can worsen existing socioeconomic inequalities, as certain jobs and industries are more susceptible to automation than others. For example, low-skilled and manual labour positions are often at higher risk of being replaced by AI-driven automation, while jobs requiring complex decision-making, creativity, and emotional intelligence are typically more resistant to automation.

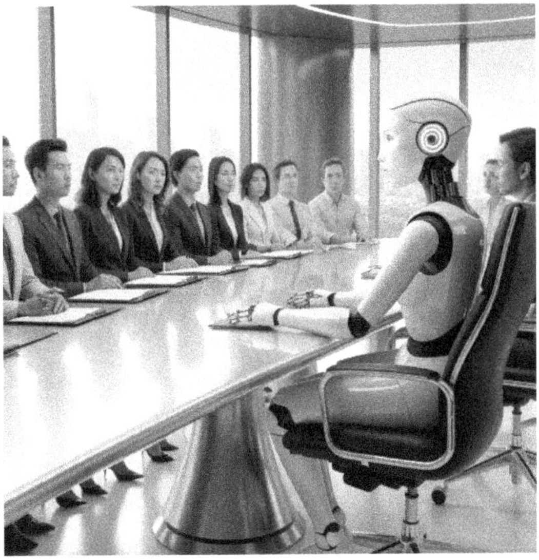

As AI advances, its role raises both collaboration opportunities and concerns over job displacement

The potential for widespread job displacement underscores the importance of proactive measures to address the impact of AI on the workforce. This includes investing in education and training programs to equip workers with the skills needed for jobs that are less susceptible to automation. Additionally, policymakers need to consider implementing policies such as job retraining initiatives, income support programs, and labour market reforms to mitigate the negative consequences of job displacement and ensure a smooth transition to an AI-driven economy.

Moreover, businesses and organizations must prioritize responsible AI deployment practices that consider the social and ethical implications of automation on the workforce. This may involve implementing strategies to upskill existing employees, fostering a culture of lifelong learning and adaptability, and exploring alternative employment opportunities within AI-driven industries.

Ultimately, while AI-driven automation has the potential to increase productivity and efficiency, addressing the challenges of job displacement requires a collaborative effort involving government, industry, academia, and civil society to ensure that the benefits of AI are shared equitably and that no one is left behind in the transition to an AI-powered future.

Example in Healthcare Context: In the medical field, job displacement due to AI automation can be illustrated by the adoption of AI-powered diagnostic systems. For instance, imagine a hospital implementing an AI system capable of analysing medical images, such as X-rays or MRI scans, to assist radiologists in detecting abnormalities or diseases. Traditionally, radiologists spend significant time and expertise examining these images to make accurate diagnoses. However, with the introduction of AI diagnostic systems, many routine tasks involved in image interpretation can be automated. AI algorithms can quickly analyse vast amounts of imaging data, identifying patterns and anomalies that may indicate the presence of a particular condition.

While AI-driven diagnostic systems can enhance efficiency and accuracy in medical imaging interpretation, they also have the potential to displace certain tasks traditionally performed by radiologists. For example, tasks such as identifying common abnormalities or screening for certain conditions may be automated by AI, reducing the amount of time radiologists need to spend on these routine tasks.

As a result, there is a possibility of job displacement for radiologists who primarily perform these tasks. While AI may augment the capabilities of radiologists and improve overall diagnostic accuracy, it may also lead to a shift in the role of radiologists towards more complex cases requiring human expertise, interpretation, and decision-making.

To address the potential job displacement in this scenario, hospitals and healthcare institutions may need to invest in training programs to upskill radiologists in areas where human expertise remains essential, such as interpreting complex imaging findings, communicating with patients, and collaborating with other healthcare professionals to develop comprehensive treatment plans.

Additionally, policymakers and healthcare organizations may need to consider implementing policies and initiatives to support displaced workers, such as job retraining programs, career counselling services, and opportunities for reemployment within the healthcare sector or other related fields.

By proactively addressing the challenges of job displacement in the medical field, stakeholders can ensure a smooth transition to an AI-driven healthcare system while preserving the crucial role of human expertise and compassion in patient care.

d) Security and privacy risks associated with AI systems are multifaceted and pose significant challenges in various domains. AI algorithms, particularly those employing machine learning techniques, rely heavily on data for training and decision-making. However, this reliance on data introduces vulnerabilities that can be exploited by malicious actors. For instance, adversarial attacks can manipulate input data to deceive AI systems, leading to incorrect or compromised outputs. Additionally, AI models themselves can be targeted for attacks, such as model inversion attacks, where attackers attempt to extract sensitive information from the model by analysing its outputs.

Furthermore, the collection and utilization of personal data by AI systems raise concerns about privacy infringement. AI algorithms often require access to large datasets, which may include sensitive information about individuals, such as health records, financial transactions, or personal preferences. If not properly managed, this data can be susceptible to breaches or unauthorized access, compromising individuals' privacy and confidentiality.

Moreover, the deployment of AI systems in various applications, such as autonomous vehicles, smart homes, and healthcare, amplifies the potential impact of security and privacy breaches. For instance, a security breach in an autonomous vehicle's AI system could lead to serious safety risks for passengers and pedestrians. Similarly, vulnerabilities in AI-driven healthcare systems could result in unauthorized access to patients' medical records or tampering with treatment recommendations, jeopardizing patient safety and trust in healthcare providers.

Addressing security and privacy risks associated with AI systems requires a multifaceted approach. This includes implementing robust cyber security measures to protect AI systems from external threats, such as encryption, authentication mechanisms, and intrusion detection systems. Additionally, organizations must adhere to stringent data protection regulations and standards to safeguard individuals' privacy rights, such as the General Data Protection Regulation (GDPR) in Europe or the Health Insurance Portability and Accountability Act (HIPAA) in the United States and proposed Digital Information Security in Healthcare Act (DISHA) in India.

Furthermore, promoting transparency and accountability in AI development and deployment is crucial for building trust and confidence among users and stakeholders. This involves conducting thorough risk assessments, auditing AI systems for vulnerabilities, and providing clear communication about data collection, usage, and security practices to users.

By prioritizing security and privacy considerations throughout the AI lifecycle, stakeholders can mitigate the risks posed by AI systems and ensure that these technologies continue to benefit society while respecting individuals' rights and safety.

Example in Healthcare Context: In the medical context, security and privacy risks associated with AI systems can be exemplified by the deployment of AI-driven electronic health record (EHR) systems. These systems store vast amounts of sensitive patient information, including medical histories, diagnoses, treatments, and laboratory results.

One security risk involves the potential for unauthorized access to EHR systems by malicious actors. If AI algorithms used for data analysis or decision support within these systems are not adequately secured, they could become targets for cyber-attacksaimed at stealing or tampering with patient data. For example, attackers may exploit vulnerabilities in AI models to gain unauthorized access to patients' medical records, compromising their privacy and confidentiality.

Moreover, the interconnected nature of healthcare systems increases the risk of data breaches. For instance, if an AI-powered diagnostic tool integrated with an EHR system is compromised, it could provide attackers with a pathway to access sensitive patient data stored in the EHR.

Additionally, the use of AI algorithms in medical imaging systems introduces privacy risks related to the handling of patient images.

For instance, AI algorithms trained on medical imaging data may inadvertently reveal identifying information about patients if not properly anonymised or secured. This could lead to unintended privacy breaches, especially if images containing personally identifiable information are shared or used for research purposes without adequate safeguards in place.

Furthermore, ongoing monitoring and auditing of AI systems are essential to detect and respond to security threats promptly. This includes conducting regular vulnerability assessments, penetration testing, and security audits to identify and address potential weaknesses in AI algorithms and systems.

By prioritizing security and privacy considerations in the development and deployment of AI-driven medical systems, healthcare organizations can safeguard patient data and maintain trust in the integrity and confidentiality of healthcare services.

e) The ethical concerns surrounding AI are multifaceted and touch upon various aspects of human society. One significant ethical concern is the potential erosion of individual autonomy when AI systems make decisions that affect people's lives without their direct involvement or consent. This raises questions about the extent to which humans should delegate decision-making authority to AI, especially in critical domains such as healthcare, criminal justice, and finance.

Furthermore, the issue of accountability becomes paramount in situations where AI systems make erroneous or biased decisions, leading to adverse outcomes for individuals or communities. Determining who bears responsibility for such decisions, whether it's the developers, deployers, or users of AI systems, poses complex ethical dilemmas and legal challenges that must be addressed to ensure fair and just outcomes.

Moreover, AI technologies can also raise concerns about the preservation of human dignity, particularly in contexts where they are used to assess, categorize, or treat individuals based on sensitive attributes such as race, gender, or socioeconomic status. Biases inherent in AI systems can perpetuate systemic inequalities and discrimination, undermining the principles of fairness, equity, and human rights.

Additionally, there are ethical considerations surrounding the use of AI in surveillance and social control, where the indiscriminate collection and analysis of data infringe upon individuals' privacy rights and civil liberties. This raises questions about the balance between security and privacy, as well as the potential for AI-powered surveillance to be abused for political repression or social manipulation.

Furthermore, the ethical implications of AI extend to issues of transparency, explainability, and consent, where individuals have the right to understand how AI systems make decisions that affect them and to provide informed consent for the collection and use of their data.

Addressing these ethical concerns requires a holistic approach that involves interdisciplinary collaboration among technologists, ethicists, policymakers, and society at large. It necessitates the development of ethical frameworks, guidelines, and regulations to ensure that AI technologies are designed, deployed, and governed in a manner that upholds human values, rights, and dignity.

By fostering ethical awareness and responsible AI practices, we can harness the potential of AI to advance human welfare and societal progress while mitigating its negative impacts on individuals and communities.

Example in Healthcare Context: In the medical context, ethical concerns surrounding AI can be illustrated by the use of AI-driven decision-making systems for patient care. For instance, imagine a scenario where an AI algorithm is deployed to assist healthcare providers in triaging patients in a hospital emergency department based on the severity of their condition.

While the AI system may offer efficiency gains by prioritizing patients who require immediate attention, ethical questions arise regarding the fairness and accuracy of its decisions. There may be concerns about whether the algorithm takes into account relevant factors beyond medical indicators, such as patients' socioeconomic status, access to healthcare resources, or cultural backgrounds, which could influence their treatment priorities.

Furthermore, if the AI algorithm is not transparent or explainable, healthcare providers and patients may lack insight into how decisions are made, raising concerns about accountability and trust. Patients may feel apprehensive about entrusting critical healthcare decisions to a system they do not fully understand, particularly if its decision-making process is opaque or biased.

Moreover, there may be ethical dilemmas regarding the allocation of scarce medical resources, such as organ transplants or intensive care unit (ICU) beds, where AI-driven algorithms are used to prioritize patients based on prognostic factors and treatment outcomes. Balancing the principles of justice, equity, and patient welfare in resource allocation decisions made by AI systems requires careful consideration of ethical guidelines and societal values.

Additionally, the use of AI in medical research and clinical trials raises ethical concerns about informed consent, privacy protection, and data ownership. Patients' health data collected for research purposes must be handled with integrity and respect for their autonomy and privacy rights, with clear protocols in place for obtaining informed consent and ensuring data security.

Addressing these ethical concerns in the medical application of AI requires robust ethical frameworks, guidelines, and governance mechanisms that prioritize patient welfare, transparency, accountability, and equity. It also necessitates ongoing dialogue and collaboration among healthcare professionals, ethicists, regulators, and patients to ensure that AI technologies are deployed in a manner that upholds ethical principles and promotes the well-being of individuals and communities.

1.1.4 Forms of AI

Artificial Intelligence encompasses a spectrum of capabilities, ranging from specialized 'weak AI,' which focuses on narrow tasks, to the theoretical 'strong AI,' which aims to replicate human-like intelligence across a broad range of domains.

i. Weak AI:

Weak AI, often referred to as narrow AI, is designed with a singular focus, tailored to excel in a predefined domain. Unlike general AI, which aims to mimic human cognitive abilities across a broad spectrum of tasks, weak AI systems operate within clearly defined parameters. These systems leverage specialized algorithms and data sets to achieve proficiency in tasks ranging from natural language processing to image recognition. Despite their limited scope, weak AI solutions have demonstrated remarkable effectiveness in various fields, including healthcare, finance, and manufacturing. In the realm of weak AI, iconic examples like IBM's Deep Blue, which famously defeated chess grandmaster Garry Kasparov in 1997, demonstrate the remarkable efficiency of specialized systems in solving singular tasks. Their ability to streamline processes, enhance decision-making, and automate routine tasks underscores their significance in contemporary technological landscapes. As advancements continue, the deployment of weak AI is anticipated to burgeon, offering targeted solutions to address specific challenges across diverse industries. In healthcare, weak AI systems have been instrumental in revolutionizing various AI algorithms can analyse medical images such as X-rays, MRIs, and CT scans with incredible precision. These systems can detect anomalies, identify potential diseases, and assist radiologists in making more accurate diagnoses. Moreover, weak AI-driven chatbots and virtual assistants are deployed in healthcare settings to provide patients with personalized medical advice, schedule appointments, and offer basic triage services.

Furthermore, weak AI is utilized in predictive analytics models that analyse patient data to forecast disease progression, identify at-risk individuals, and recommend personalized treatment plans. These algorithms sift through vast amounts of patient information, including medical records, genetic data, and lifestyle factors, to generate actionable insights for healthcare providers.

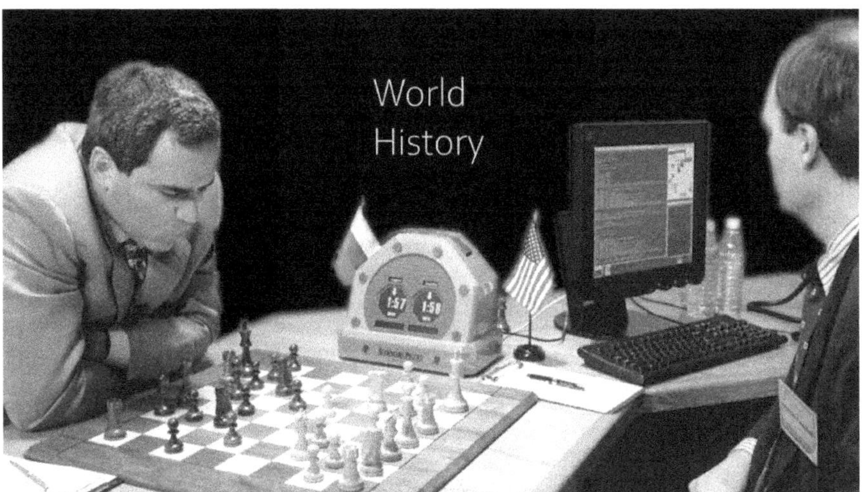

The Kasparov-Deep Blue match showcased AI's potential while challenging human supremacy in strategic thought

ii. Strong AI:

Strong AI, also known as artificial general intelligence (AGI), represents the pinnacle of artificial intelligence research and development. Unlike weak AI, which is specialized in solving specific tasks, strong AI aims to replicate the breadth and depth of human intelligence across a wide range of domains. Creating strong AI is an immensely challenging endeavour due to the complexity of human cognition and the myriad of skills and abilities it encompasses. AGI systems are designed to not only perform tasks but also to understand, learn, and adapt to new situations autonomously, exhibiting cognitive capabilities akin to those of humans.

The development of strong AI requires breakthroughs in various fields, including machine learning, cognitive science, neuroscience, and philosophy. Researchers seek to imbue AGI systems with the capacity for abstract reasoning, creativity, emotional intelligence, and ethical decision-making, among other human-like attributes. Achieving true strong AI entails creating machines that can comprehend natural language, engage in meaningful conversation, perceive the world through sensory inputs, and navigate complex social dynamics.

While significant progress has been made in AI research, achieving strong AI remains an elusive goal, with many technical, ethical, and philosophical challenges yet to be overcome. However, the pursuit of strong AI holds immense promise for advancing humanity's understanding of intelligence, consciousness, and the nature of mind. If successful, strong AI could revolutionize virtually every aspect of human society, from healthcare and education to economics and governance, ushering in a new era of unprecedented possibilities and challenges.

1.2 Why AI booming

The AI technology is a bit old and stagnated decades before getting boomed recently. Despite early promise, the technology struggled to achieve widespread adoption due to limitations in computing power, algorithmic complexity, and the availability of large-scale data etc. During that time, AI remained largely confined to academic research labs and specialized applications, with mainstream integration limited by practical constraints and technological hurdles. As computing technology continued to advance and data generation increased exponentially, the stage was set for a paradigm shift in AI capabilities.

The boom in AI can be attributed to several factors that have converged to create a conducive environment for its rapid development and adoption. Some key reasons include:

1. Advancements in Technology: Significant advancements in hardware, such as Graphics Processing Units (GPUs), have enhanced the processing power available for AI tasks, enabling more complex and sophisticated algorithms to be executed efficiently. Moreover, the miniaturization of hardware components, coupled with increased energy efficiency, has facilitated the development of AI-powered devices with greater mobility and autonomy. These advancements have paved the way for the proliferation of AI applications in areas such as robotics, Internet of Things (IoT) devices, and wearable technology.

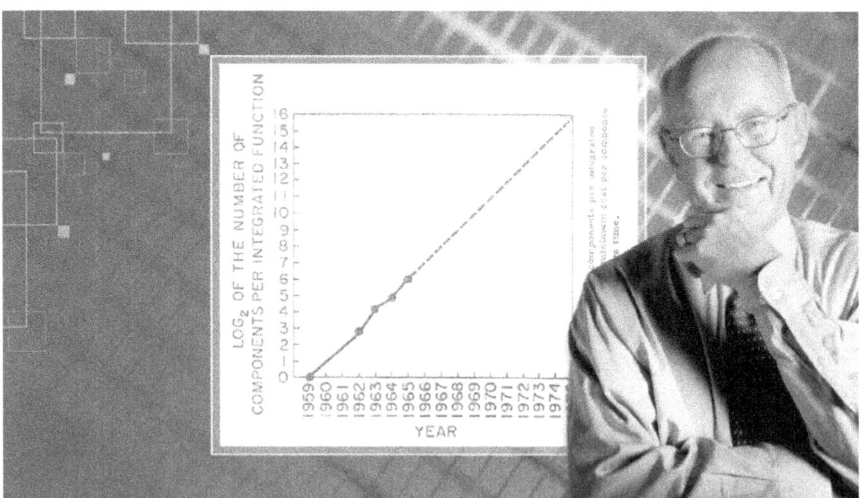

Gordon Moore

Additionally, innovations in specialized hardware accelerators, such as Tensor Processing Units (TPUs) and Field-Programmable Gate Arrays (FPGAs), have been tailored to meet the unique computational requirements of AI workloads. These dedicated processing units enable faster inference and training times, making AI systems more responsive and efficient. Moore's Law, which has governed the exponential increase in computing power over several decades, has been a driving force behind the advancements in hardware that have fuelled the recent boom in AI. Moore's Law, named after Intel co-founder Gordon Moore, is the observation that the number of transistors on a microchip doubles approximately every two years, leading to a doubling of computational power. This empirical observation has been a guiding principle in the semiconductor industry for decades, driving continuous advancements in computing technology. The continuous miniaturization of transistors and the increasing density of integrated circuits have enabled processors to become smaller, faster, and more energy-efficient. This relentless progress in semiconductor technology has provided the foundation for the development of GPUs, TPUs, and other specialized hardware accelerators optimized for AI workloads. By adhering to Moore's Law, manufacturers have been able to consistently deliver chips with greater computational capabilities, allowing AI researchers and developers to tackle increasingly complex problems and scale their solutions more effectively.

Furthermore, advancements in quantum computing hold the promise of revolutionizing AI by exponentially increasing processing speeds and tackling complex optimization problems that are currently beyond the reach of classical computers. While still in the early stages of development, the potential impact of quantum computing on AI cannot be overstated.

These advancements have not only enabled the execution of more complex algorithms but have also fuelled innovation across diverse application domains, driving the recent boom in AI.

2. Big Data: Big data refers to the large volume, variety, and velocity of data that inundates organizations on a daily basis. This data comes from various sources such as business transactions, social media interactions, sensors, and other digital activities. Big data is characterized by its size, complexity, and speed at which it is generated, making it difficult to process and analyse using traditional database management tools. The massive amount of data is made possible by several factors:

a) Digital Transformation: The digitization of various aspects of life, including business operations, communication, entertainment, and healthcare, has led to the generation of vast amounts of data.

b) Internet Usage: The widespread use of the internet, coupled with the proliferation of connected devices, has resulted in a constant stream of data being produced from online activities such as browsing, shopping, streaming, and social networking.

c) Sensor Technology: The deployment of sensors in various environments, including manufacturing facilities, vehicles, infrastructure, and wearable devices, generates continuous streams of data about the physical world.

d) Social Media: Platforms like Meta, X formally known as Twitter, Instagram, and LinkedIn generate enormous volumes of data through user interactions, posts, likes, shares, comments, and other activities.

e) E-commerce: Online shopping platforms collect vast amounts of data on customer behaviour, preferences, purchase history, and interactions, contributing to the big data ecosystem.

f) IoT Devices: The Internet of Things (IoT) encompasses a wide range of devices embedded with sensors and connected to the internet, generating data on everything from energy consumption and environmental conditions to health metrics and vehicle performance.

g) Data Replication and Sharing: Data is often replicated across multiple systems for redundancy, shared between organizations for collaborative purposes, and collected from third-party sources through APIs, contributing to the accumulation of massive datasets.

The availability of massive amounts of data has played a crucial role in training and improving AI models. With more data, AI systems can learn and generalize better, leading to more accurate predictions and outcomes. The diversity and richness of big data sources have enabled AI systems to gain deeper insights into complex patterns and relationships, enhancing their ability to make informed decisions across a wide range of domains. Additionally, big data has facilitated the development of more robust and adaptable AI models through techniques such as transfer learning, where knowledge gained from one dataset can be applied to related tasks or domains with limited labelled data. Moreover, the availability of big data has spurred advancements in data pre-processing, feature engineering, and data augmentation techniques, enabling AI researchers to extract meaningful information from noisy or incomplete datasets and improve the overall performance of their models.

3. Improved Algorithms: Researchers and developers have continually refined and developed new algorithms for machine learning and deep learning. This has led to improved model performance, better understanding of data, and the ability to solve more complex problems. The roots of modern AI can be traced back to the mid-20th century, with foundational algorithms such as perceptions and decision trees laying the groundwork for subsequent developments. However, it was the advent of neural networks and the backpropagation algorithm in the 1980s that sparked renewed interest in AI research. Despite initial limitations, these early algorithms paved the way for future breakthroughs by demonstrating the potential of learning algorithms to mimic human cognitive processes.

a) Breakthroughs in Machine Learning Algorithms: The turn of the millennium witnessed a renaissance in machine learning, fuelled by advancements in algorithms such as support vector machines (SVMs), random forests, and gradient boosting. These algorithms enabled more robust pattern recognition and predictive modelling, leading to applications in areas such as finance, healthcare, and marketing. Moreover, the rise of deep learning algorithms, particularly convolutional neural networks (CNNs) and recurrent neural networks (RNNs), revolutionized fields like computer vision, speech recognition, and natural language processing.

b) Impact on Natural Language Processing: One of the most significant areas influenced by improved algorithms is natural language processing (NLP). Traditional approaches to NLP relied on handcrafted rules and heuristics, limiting their scalability and performance. However, the advent of deep learning algorithms, coupled with the availability of large-scale datasets, has led to remarkable progress in tasks such as sentiment analysis, machine translation, and question answering. Transformer-based models like BERT and GPT have achieved state-of-the-art results across various NLP benchmarks, showcasing the power of advanced algorithms in understanding and generating human language.

c) Revolutionizing Computer Vision: Computer vision is another domain that has witnessed a paradigm shift due to improved algorithms. Early computer vision systems struggled with image understanding and object recognition tasks, often relying on handcrafted features and shallow learning models. With the rise of deep learning algorithms, particularly CNNs, researchers achieved unprecedented accuracy in tasks such as image classification, object detection, and image segmentation. Applications of computer vision algorithms range from autonomous vehicles and medical imaging to augmented reality and facial recognition systems.

d) Advancements in Reinforcement Learning: Reinforcement learning (RL) has emerged as a powerful paradigm for training intelligent agents to interact with dynamic environments. Improved algorithms in RL, such as deep Q-learning and policy gradient methods, have led to significant breakthroughs in tasks ranging from game playing to robotics. AlphaGo's victory over human Go champions and OpenAI's success in mastering complex video games demonstrate the effectiveness of advanced algorithms in learning complex behaviours through trial and error.

4. Increased Computational Power: The availability of high-performance computing resources, both in terms of hardware and cloud services, has made it easier for organizations and researchers to experiment with and deploy AI solutions at scale.

Machine learning and deep learning, subfields of AI, have witnessed exponential growth in recent years, thanks in large part to increased computational power. Training deep neural networks, which require massive amounts of computational resources, has become feasible at scale due to advancements in parallel computing and distributed systems. As a result, researchers can now tackle larger datasets, train more complex models, and achieve unprecedented levels of accuracy in tasks such as image recognition, natural language processing, and speech synthesis. Moreover, the availability of cloud computing services and specialized hardware platforms has democratized access to high-performance computing, empowering researchers and developers worldwide to innovate and collaborate on AI projects. Additionally, the increased computational power has facilitated the development of sophisticated optimization techniques and algorithms, allowing AI systems to efficiently process and analyse vast amounts of data. This capability is particularly crucial in fields such as predictive analytics, where AI models can identify patterns and trends within complex datasets to make accurate forecasts and recommendations. Furthermore, increased computational power is driving advancements in reinforcement learning, a branch of AI focused on training agents to make sequential decisions through interaction with an environment. Moreover, the combination of increased computational power and AI algorithms is revolutionizing personalized user experiences across various digital platforms.

5. Open Source Communities: The exponential growth of Artificial Intelligence owes much to the collaborative efforts of open source communities. The open-source nature of many AI frameworks and libraries, such as TensorFlow, PyTorch and scikit-learn has fostered collaboration and knowledge sharing among researchers and developers. This has accelerated the pace of innovation in the field. These frameworks offer a wide range of functionalities, from basic algorithms and optimization techniques to advanced deep learning architectures and pre-trained models. By making these tools freely available and accessible, open source initiatives have lowered barriers to entry and empowered researchers and developers to explore new ideas, algorithms, and applications. Furthermore, open source communities have played a vital role in advancing AI research through collaborative projects and initiatives. Platforms like GitHub and GitLab provide infrastructure for hosting, sharing, and collaborating on code repositories, enabling distributed teams to work together seamlessly. Organisation such as OpenAI, DeepMind, and the Allen Institute for AI release research code and datasets under open source licenses, facilitating reproducibility, peer review, and knowledge dissemination within the scientific community. By providing free and open-source software tools, libraries, and resources, these communities have levelled the playing field, enabling individuals and organizations of all sizes to leverage AI for innovation and problem-solving. By welcoming contributions from developers of diverse backgrounds, experiences, and expertise, open source projects benefit from a broad range of perspectives and insights. This diversity enriches the quality of AI solutions, enhances robustness and reliability, and ensures that AI technologies reflect the needs and values of society as a whole. Furthermore, open source initiatives facilitate interoperability and compatibility between different AI tools

and platforms, enabling seamless integration and deployment of AI solutions. This interoperability fosters an ecosystem of complementary technologies and services, driving innovation and enabling cross-disciplinary collaborations. For example, open source projects like ONNX (Open Neural Network Exchange) enable interoperability between different deep learning frameworks, allowing developers to train models in one framework and deploy them in another.

6. Investments and Funding: There has been a significant increase in investments and funding for AI research and development. Governments, private companies, and venture capitalists recognize the potential of AI and are investing in projects and startups working in this space. This surge in financial support has propelled the AI ecosystem forward, driving innovation, fostering collaboration, and fuelling the rapid expansion of AI-driven solutions.

Several factors have contributed to the exponential rise in investments and funding for AI research and development

a) Technological Advancements: Breakthroughs in AI algorithms, machine learning techniques, and computational power have unlocked new possibilities, making AI more capable, efficient, and accessible than ever before. These advancements have spurred investor confidence in the potential of AI to drive innovation and create value across multiple domains.

b) Demonstrated Success Stories: High-profile successes in AI applications, such as natural language processing, computer vision, and autonomous vehicles, have captured the imagination of investors and demonstrated the tangible impact of AI on business outcomes. These success stories have validated the business case for AI investments and fuelled interest from both traditional and non-traditional investors.

c) Market Opportunities: The proliferation of data, coupled with advances in data collection, storage, and processing technologies, has created a fertile ground for AI-driven solutions. Industries ranging from healthcare and finance to manufacturing and transportation are actively seeking AI-powered tools and services to optimize operations, enhance decision-making, and gain competitive advantages in the marketplace.

d) Regulatory Support: Governments around the world have recognized the strategic importance of AI and have introduced policies and initiatives to support its development. From funding research grants and establishing AI hubs to promoting ethical guidelines and standards, regulatory support has provided a conducive environment for AI investments to thrive.

e) Global Competition: The intensifying global competition in AI leadership has incentivized countries, companies, and investors to ramp up their investments in AI research and development. As AI increasingly becomes a cornerstone of economic competitiveness and national security, stakeholders are vying for leadership positions in the AI landscape, driving investment flows and innovation cycles.

Sources of Funding: Investments in AI research and development come from diverse sources, including:

a) Government Funding: Governments allocate resources to support AI research and development through grants, contracts, and public-private partnerships. These investments aim to advance scientific knowledge, promote technological innovation, and address societal challenges through AI-driven solutions.

b) Corporate Investments: Private companies across various industries invest in AI research and development to drive business growth, enhance competitiveness, and capitalize on emerging market opportunities. Tech giants like Google, Microsoft, and Amazon are leading the charge in AI investments, leveraging their expertise, resources, and data assets to develop AI-powered products and services.

c) Venture Capital: Venture capitalists and angel investors provide funding to AI start-ups and early-stage companies in exchange for equity stakes. These investments fuel innovation, enable market entry, and support entrepreneurial ventures in developing AI-driven solutions across diverse domains.

d) Academic Institutions: Universities and research institutions conduct fundamental research in AI and receive funding from government grants, industry partnerships, and philanthropic donations. These investments contribute to the advancement of scientific knowledge, the training of future AI professionals, and the dissemination of research findings to the broader community.

e) International Collaboration: Multinational organizations, consortia, and research networks collaborate on AI research and development initiatives, pooling resources, expertise, and data to tackle global challenges and accelerate progress in AI technologies. These collaborative efforts facilitate knowledge exchange, technology transfer, and capacity building across borders.

In addition to the factors mentioned above, the following elements have also contributed to catalysing the AI boom.

a) Integration into Various Industries: AI has demonstrated its ability to bring value across a wide range of industries, including healthcare, finance, manufacturing, and more. This success has led to increased interest and adoption as businesses seek to leverage AI for competitive advantage.

b) Enhanced User Experience: AI-powered applications have improved user experiences in various domains, such as natural language processing, image recognition, and recommendation systems. This has led to increased consumer demand and acceptance of AI technologies.

c) Automation and Efficiency: Businesses are adopting AI to automate repetitive tasks, enhance efficiency, and reduce operational costs. AI-driven automation is particularly attractive in industries where large-scale data processing and decision-making are critical.

d) Ethical and Social Considerations: As AI technologies mature, there is also a growing awareness of ethical considerations, responsible AI development, and the need to address bias and fairness. This has led to a more conscientious approach to AI research and deployment.

Chapter
02

COMMON TECHNIQUES USED IN AI

Common techniques used in artificial intelligence encompass a broad array of methodologies aimed at enabling machines to perform tasks that typically require human intelligence. These techniques leverage various algorithms, models, and approaches to simulate cognitive functions, learn from data, and make decisions. Here's an overview of some of the most prevalent techniques used in AI:

2.1 Machine Learning

Machine learning is a subset of artificial intelligence focus on developing algorithms and statistical models which allow computers to learn from data and make predictions or decisions its own, without explicit programming. Essentially, it involves training machines to recognize patterns in data and enhance their performance over time, enabling them to sense trends, forecast outcomes, and address complex problems in various fields. Machine learning is commonly classified into three primary categories: Supervised Learning, Unsupervised Learning, and Reinforcement Learning.

2.1.1 Supervised Learning

Definition: In supervised learning, the algorithm learns from a labelled dataset, where each input data point is associated with a corresponding output label. The aim is for the algorithm to understand the relationship between inputs and outputs

Process: During training, the algorithm adjusts its parameters to minimize the difference between its predicted outputs and the true labels in the training data.

Example: Using patient data (features like age, genetic markers, lifestyle factors) labelled with disease outcomes (presence or absence of a disease), a model can be trained to predict the risk of developing a particular disease, such as diabetes or cancer.

Working of Supervised Learning

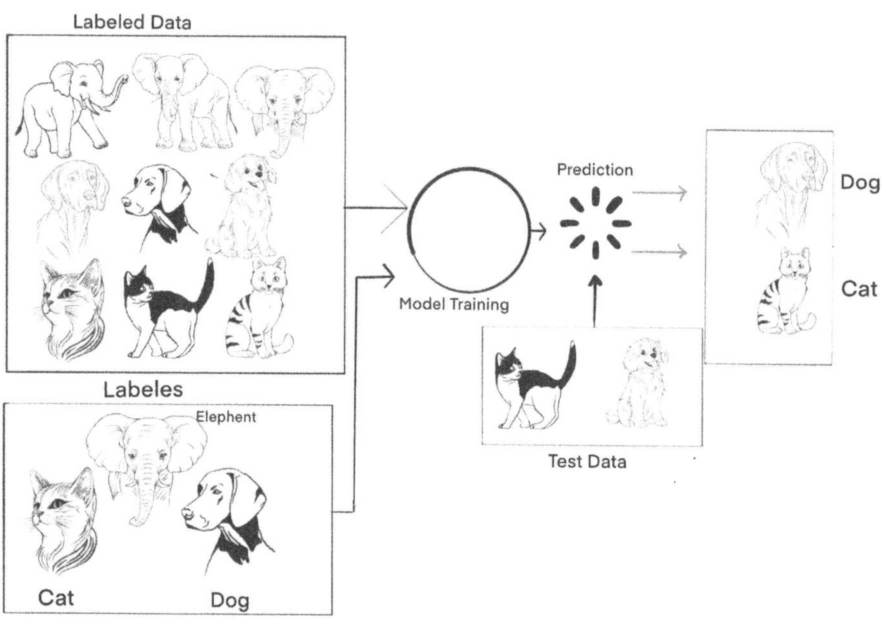

Supervised Learning

Suppose we have a dataset of different animals like, cat, dog and elephant. Initially we need to train the model for each animal. We will teach the model how a cat looks like, how a dog looks like and how an elephant looks like.

Now, after teaching (training), we want to conduct a test for the model whether our model learned well enough to identify any image of the trained animals using the test set. This test set will be a completely different set of animals from the training set. If the machine is already trained well on features of different animals then it can classify the animals to the category of cat, dog and elephant on the bases of these unique features and predicts the output. With a comparison of machine output with a known test data output we can determine the accuracy of the model. If there is a mismatch between the predicted output and actual output from the model, then we need to have further adjustment of the model using parameters like weight and bias.

Types of supervised Machine learning Algorithms

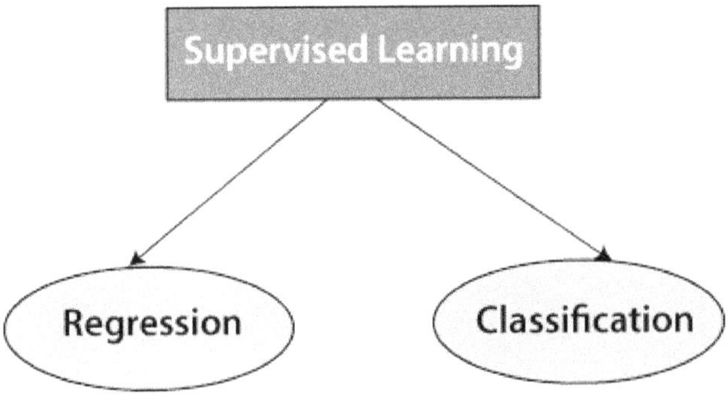

1. Regression

Regression algorithms are applied when there is a relationship between the input and output variables. They are used to predict continuous variables, such as weather forecasts, housing prices etc. Below are some popular regression algorithms which come under supervised learning:

- Linear Regression
- Regression Trees
- Non-Linear Regression
- Bayesian Linear Regression
- Polynomial Regression

2. Classification

Classification algorithms are employed when the output variable is categorical, meaning it belongs to distinct classes such as Pass-Fail, True-False, and Accept-Reject-etc. Here are some well-known classification algorithms that fall under supervised learning.

- Random Forest
- Decision Trees
- Logistic Regression
- Support vector Machines

Advantages of Supervised learning

- Supervised learning allows the model to predict outcomes based on previous experiences.
- This type of model helps address various real-world issues, such as fraud detection and spam filtering.
- With supervised learning, we can precisely identify the classes of objects.

Disadvantages of supervised learning

- Supervised learning models are not well-suited for managing highly complex tasks.
- Supervised learning models may struggle to generalize well if the test data distribution is significantly different from the training data distribution
- Training required lots of computation times.
- In supervised learning, a sufficient understanding of the object classes is required.

2.1.2 Unsupervised Learning

Definition: Unsupervised learning involves training a model on data without explicit output labels. The algorithm explores the inherent structure and patterns within the data.

Process: Common techniques include clustering (grouping similar data points together) and dimensionality reduction (simplifying the data while retaining important information).

Example: Anomaly detection in medical devices or patient monitoring systems. Consider a scenario where continuous physiological data, such as heart rate, blood pressure, and oxygen saturation levels, are collected from patients using wearable devices or bedside monitors in a hospital. By applying unsupervised learning algorithms, patterns of normal behaviour can be learned without requiring labelled instances of anomalies.

Working of Unsupervised Learning

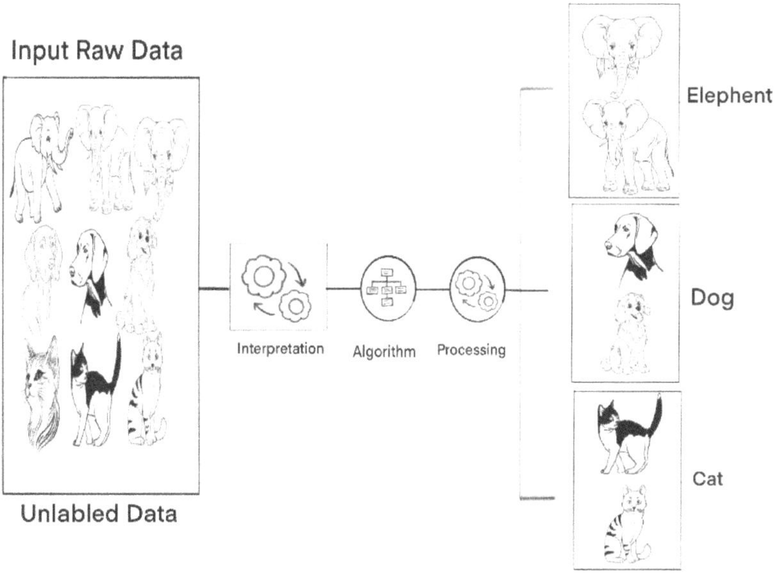

Unsupervised Learning

In this scenario, we start with unlabelled input data, meaning it is neither categorized nor paired with corresponding outputs. This unlabelled data is fed into a machine learning model for training. Initially, the model analyses the raw data to uncover hidden patterns and then applies appropriate algorithms such as k-means clustering or Decision trees.

Once the suitable algorithm is applied, it categorizes the data objects into groups based on their similarities and differences.

Types of Unsupervised Learning Algorithm:

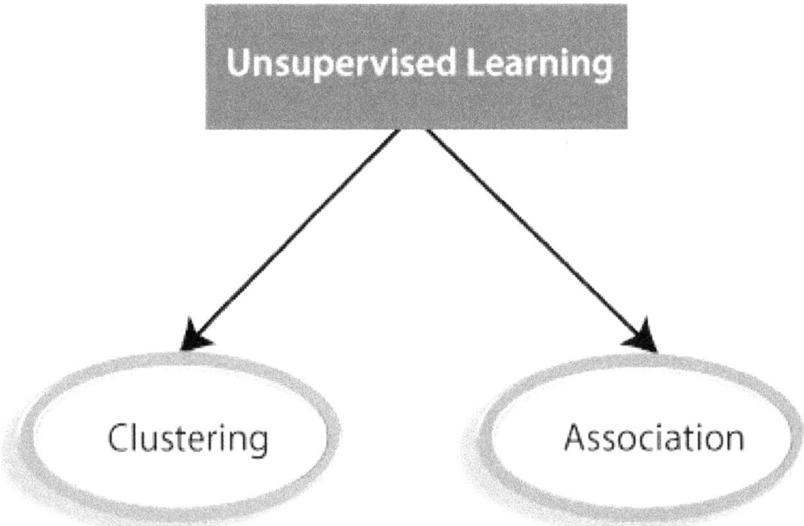

1. Clustering: Clustering is a technique for grouping objects into clusters where objects with the most similarities are placed in the same group, and have fewer or no similarities with objects in other groups. Cluster analysis identifies commonalities among data objects and categorizes them based on the presence or absence of these commonalities.
2. Association: An association rule is an unsupervised learning method used to identify relationships between variables in large databases. It discovers sets of items that frequently appear together in the dataset. Association rules can enhance marketing strategies, such as identifying that customers who purchase item X (e.g., bread) are also likely to buy item Y (e.g., butter or jam). A common application of association rules is Market Basket Analysis.

Advantages of Unsupervised Learning

- Unsupervised learning is utilized for more complex tasks compared to supervised learning because it does not require labelled input data.
- Unsupervised learning is often preferred because obtaining unlabelled data is generally easier than acquiring labelled data.
- Unsupervised learning algorithms can handle large volumes of data more efficiently since they do not require the extensive and often time-consuming process of labelling.

Disadvantages of Unsupervised Learning

- Unsupervised learning is inherently more challenging than supervised learning because it lacks corresponding output data.
- The outcomes of unsupervised learning algorithms may be less accurate since the input data is unlabelled and the algorithms do not have predefined outputs.
- While unsupervised learning can handle large datasets, some algorithms may struggle with very large or complex datasets due to computational limitations.

2.1.3 Reinforcement Learning

Definition: Reinforcement learning involves training an agent to make decisions within an environment by receiving feedback in the form of rewards or penalties. The agent learns to perform actions that maximize the cumulative reward over time.

Process: The agent explores the environment, takes actions, receives feedback, and adjusts its strategy based on the rewards it receives.

Example: Reinforcement learning (RL) can be applied to develop adaptive treatment strategies that dynamically adjust medical interventions based on patient responses and feedback over time. This approach aims to optimize treatment outcomes while minimizing adverse effects and resource utilization.

Core Characteristics of Reinforcement Learning

- The environment is stochastic, and the agent needs to explore it to reach to get the maximum positive reward
- It operates on a trial-and-error basis.
- The agent decides its next action and changes states based on the feedback from the previous action.
- The agent may receive rewards with a delay.
- In reinforcement learning, the agent is not given instructions about the environment or the actions to take.
- The environment is unpredictable, and the agent must explore it to achieve the maximum possible reward.

2.2 Deep Learning

Definition: Deep learning is a subset of machine learning that involves artificial neural networks with multiple layers (deep neural networks). These networks can automatically learn hierarchical representations of data.

Process: Deep learning models learn to extract features from data through multiple layers of interconnected nodes (neurons).

Example: Medical Image Analysis

Deep learning, particularly convolution neural networks (CNNs), is extensively used in medical image analysis. For instance, in radiology, CNNs can analyse X-rays, MRIs, or CT scans to detect abnormalities like tumours, fractures, or lesions. This technology enhances diagnostic accuracy and efficiency by automating the interpretation of medical images, assisting radiologists in identifying critical findings.

2.2.1 Core Concepts of Deep Learning

Before exploring the complexities of deep learning algorithms and their uses, it's crucial to grasp the fundamental concepts that underpin this groundbreaking technology.

Neural networks

Neural networks are the foundation of deep learning, modelled after the human brain. These networks are made up of interconnected nodes, or "neurons," that collaboratively process information and make decisions. Similar to how the brain has various regions for different tasks, a neural network features layers assigned to specific functions. A neural network is considered "deep" due to the number of layers it contains between the input and output. With multiple layers, a deep neural network can learn more intricate features and make more accurate predictions.

Activation Function

In a neural network, an activation function is a crucial step that determines what signal should be passed forward to the next layer of the network. Think of it as a decision-making gate that processes the input and decides if it should be activated (passed on) or not. It is a mathematical function that determines the output of a neuron. After a neuron processes its inputs and computes a weighted sum, the activation function is applied to this sum to introduce non-linearity into the network. This non-linearity allows the network to model complex patterns and relationships in the data.

2.2.2 How Deep Learning Works

Deep learning uses feature extraction to recognize similar attributes linked to the same label and then applies decision boundaries to determine which features accurately correspond to each label. For example, in a cats and dogs classification task, deep learning models extract information such as eyes, facial features, and body shape, categorizing them into two distinct classes. A deep learning model comprises deep neural networks. While a simple neural network includes an input layer, a hidden layer, and an output layer, deep learning models feature multiple hidden layers. The addition of these extra layers enhances the model's accuracy.

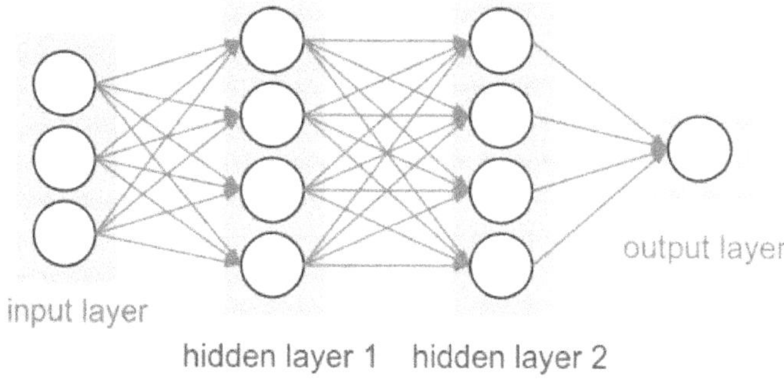

Simple Neural Network

The input layers hold raw data and pass it on to the nodes in the hidden layers. The nodes in the hidden layers classify the data points based on broader target information, progressively narrowing down the target value with each subsequent layer to achieve accurate predictions. The output layer then utilizes the information from the hidden layers to choose the most likely label. For instance, in our scenario, it accurately identifies an image as a dog rather than a cat.

2.3 Natural Language Processing

Definition: NLP involves the interaction between computers and human language. It includes tasks such as language understanding, sentiment analysis, and language generation.

Process: Techniques include tokenization, parsing, and machine learning approaches to understand and generate human language.

Example: Electronic Health Record (EHR) Analysis

Natural language processing techniques are applied in the medical field to analyse unstructured electronic health record (EHR) text data. For example, named entity recognition (NER) can extract essential entities such as patient names, medications, diseases, and treatment procedures from clinical notes. This facilitates efficient information retrieval and enables automated data-driven decision-making in healthcare settings.

2.3.1 Components of NLP

Natural Language Processing encompasses two primary components: Natural Language Understanding (NLU) and Natural Language Generation (NLG). These components work together to enable machines to interact with human language in a meaningful way.

1. Natural Language Understanding (NLU)

Natural Language Understanding (NLU) is the component that allows machines to comprehend and analyze human language. By extracting metadata from content, NLU helps in interpreting the context and meaning of the text. The key elements of metadata include concepts, entities, keywords, emotions, relationships, and semantic roles.

2. Natural Language Generation (NLG)

Natural Language Generation (NLG) is the component responsible for converting computerized data into natural language. It acts as a translator, enabling machines to produce human-like text based on the data they process.

2.3.2 Applications of NLP

Natural Language Processing has broad applications across various fields, transforming how we interact with technology and data. Here are some key applications of NLP:

1. Text Classification

NLP is used to categorize text into predefined categories, such as spam detection in emails, sentiment analysis of social media posts, and topic classification in news articles. This helps in organizing and managing large volumes of text data efficiently.

2. Machine Translation

NLP powers machine translation systems, such as Google Translate, enabling the automatic translation of text from one language to another. This application breaks down language barriers and facilitates global communication.

3. Sentiment Analysis

NLP algorithms analyze text to determine the sentiment expressed, whether positive, negative, or neutral. This is widely used in social media monitoring, customer feedback analysis, and market research to understand public opinion and customer satisfaction.

4. Chatbots and Virtual Assistants

NLP enables chatbots and virtual assistants, like Siri, Alexa, and Google Assistant, to understand and respond to user queries in natural language. These systems provide customer support, manage tasks, and offer personalized assistance, enhancing user experience.

5. Information Retrieval

NLP improves search engines by understanding the context and intent behind user queries, providing more relevant and accurate search results. It is also used in specialized databases, such as legal and medical information retrieval systems.

6. Named Entity Recognition (NER)

NLP identifies and classifies named entities, such as people, organizations, locations, dates, and other proper nouns, within text. This is useful for information extraction, data organization, and enhancing search functionalities.

7. Text Summarization

NLP algorithms generate concise summaries of longer texts, making it easier to grasp the main points quickly. This is particularly useful for news aggregation, research paper summaries, and summarizing lengthy documents.

8. Speech Recognition

NLP, combined with speech recognition technology, converts spoken language into text. This is widely used in transcription services, voice-activated assistants, and automated customer service systems.

9. Question Answering Systems

NLP powers question answering systems that automatically respond to questions posed by users in natural language. These systems are used in customer support, educational platforms, and information retrieval systems.

10. Text Generation

NLP enables the generation of human-like text, which is used in applications such as content creation, automated report writing, and creative writing assistance.

2.4 Computer Vision

Definition: Computer vision enables machines to interpret and make decisions based on visual data, such as images or videos.

Process: Techniques include image recognition, object detection, and image segmentation using deep learning models.

Example: Histopathology Image Analysis

Computer vision techniques, including image segmentation, are utilized in histopathology image analysis. Histopathology slides contain extensive tissue data, and image segmentation can partition different cell types, enabling automated analysis for cancer diagnosis and grading. By accurately identifying and quantifying cellular structures, computer vision assists pathologists in diagnosing diseases and assessing prognosis.

2.4.1 How does Computer Vision Work?

While computer vision mimics how human eyes and the brain work together, understanding how the human brain performs visual object recognition remains one of the most significant challenges for IT professionals. Fundamentally, computer vision revolves around pattern recognition, which involves training machine systems to understand visual data like images and videos.

To begin, machines are fed a large amount of labelled visual data for training purposes. This labelled data allows the machine to analyse various patterns in the data points and associate them with the corresponding labels. For example, in the healthcare context, if we provide millions of labelled images of lung X-rays, the computer learns by analysing each image's features, such as shapes, textures, and anomalies. Through this process, it identifies patterns specific to conditions like pneumonia and creates a model. Consequently, this computer vision model can accurately determine whether an X-ray image shows signs of pneumonia for any given input image.

Chapter 03

EMERGING FRONTIERS IN AI TECHNOLOGIES

The field of Artificial Intelligence is rapidly evolving, with new breakthroughs and applications emerging at an unprecedented pace. These advancements are transforming industries, enhancing human capabilities, and reshaping the future. As we delve into the forefront of AI technologies, it's essential to understand the key areas driving this transformation. Here are some of the most exciting and promising frontiers in AI today:

3.1 Explainable AI (XAI)

Explainable AI (XAI) is a branch of artificial intelligence that focuses on making the decision-making processes of AI models understandable to humans. It involves the development of methods and techniques that allow users to comprehend and trust the outputs of machine learning and AI systems. XAI aims to provide clear, interpretable explanations for how and why AI models make certain predictions or decisions, ensuring that these processes are transparent, fair, and accountable. This is particularly important in fields where understanding the rationale behind AI decisions is crucial, such as healthcare, finance, and legal domains.

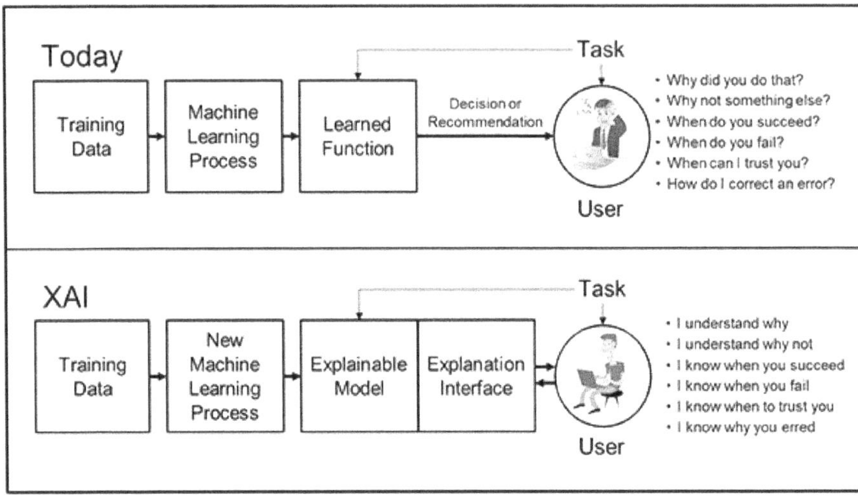

Explainable Artificial Intelligence Concept

3.1.1 Relevance of Explainable AI

The necessity for explainable AI stems from the inherent complexity and opacity of traditional machine learning models, which are often challenging to understand and interpret. These models function as black boxes, making predictions based on input data without revealing the rationale behind their outputs. This lack of transparency and interpretability poses significant limitations, leading to various problems and challenges.

One major issue with traditional machine learning models is the difficulty in establishing trust and verification. Their opaque and inscrutable nature makes it hard for humans to comprehend how these models operate and arrive at their predictions. This lack of understanding can undermine trust and hinder the adoption and deployment of such models, as people may be reluctant to rely on systems they cannot fully grasp.

In summary, the need for explainable AI arises from the limitations and challenges posed by traditional machine learning models and the demand for more transparent and interpretable models that are trustworthy, fair, and accountable. Explainable AI methods seek to overcome these challenges by providing machine learning models that offer greater transparency and interpretability, thereby enhancing human understanding and trust.

3.1.2 Benefits of explainable AI

Explainable AI offers several significant advantages, making it an essential component in the deployment and adoption of AI technologies:

1. Increased Trust and Confidence: By providing clear and understandable explanations of AI decisions, XAI helps build trust among users. When users can see how and why a decision was made, they are more likely to have confidence in the system.
2. Enhanced Accountability: XAI allows for better accountability by making it possible to trace the decision-making process of AI models. This is crucial in ensuring that AI systems are used responsibly and ethically.
3. Improved Debugging and Maintenance: Understanding the inner workings of AI models makes it easier to identify and correct errors. Developers can use XAI tools to debug and refine their models, leading to more accurate and reliable AI systems.
4. Detection and Mitigation of Bias: XAI helps in identifying biases within AI models, promoting fairness and preventing discriminatory outcomes. This is particularly important in applications that impact people's lives, such as hiring, lending, and law enforcement.
5. Regulatory Compliance: Many industries are subject to regulations that require transparency in decision-making processes. XAI assists organizations in meeting these legal and regulatory requirements, thereby avoiding potential legal issues.
6. Enhanced User Experience: By making AI systems more transparent, XAI improves the overall user experience. Users are more likely to engage with and rely on AI systems when they understand how decisions are made.

7. Better Adoption and Integration: The transparency provided by XAI facilitates the integration of AI systems into existing processes. When stakeholders understand and trust the technology, they are more likely to support its implementation and use.
8. Facilitates Ethical AI Development: XAI supports the development of ethical AI by ensuring that the decision-making processes are transparent and understandable. This helps in aligning AI systems with human values and societal norms.
9. Supports Complex Decision-Making: In fields such as healthcare and finance, where decisions can have significant consequences, XAI provides the necessary insights to support complex decision-making processes. It ensures that AI recommendations are based on sound reasoning and can be trusted by professionals.

3.2 Generative AI

Generative AI, a subset of artificial intelligence, involves algorithms that can generate new content, whether it is text, images, audio, or even video. Progress in large language models (LLMs) has fueled the evolution of Generative AI. These models are designed to understand patterns in existing data and then use this understanding to create new data with similar characteristics.

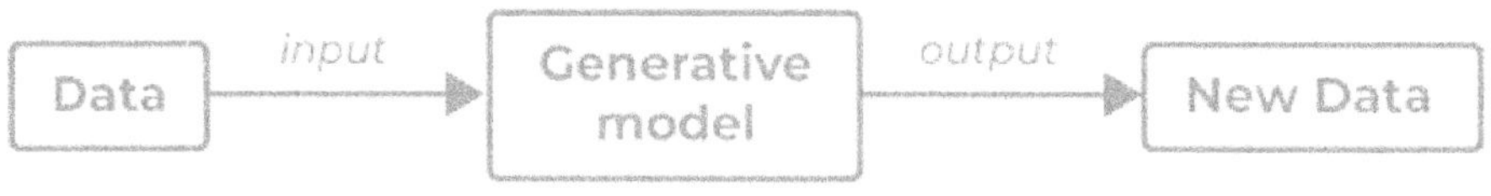

Working of Generative Model

Examples of generative AI

ChatGPT: Generative artificial intelligence created by OpenAI, a Microsoft-backed, profit-capped company. Leveraging its advanced natural language processing capabilities, ChatGPT can engage in meaningful conversations, answer complex queries, and generate coherent and contextually appropriate responses. Its versatility makes it a valuable tool across various domains, including customer support, content creation, healthcare, and research.

DALL-E: This is a generative artificial intelligence model developed by OpenAI that creates images from textual descriptions. It leverages the principles of OpenAI's advanced large language model, to understand and process text, but instead of generating text-based responses, DALL-E generates high-quality images.

Google Gemini: Google Gemini is a groundbreaking AI model developed by Google Deep Mind. It represents a significant advancement in artificial intelligence, surpassing its predecessor, Bard, in terms of capabilities and versatility.

Generative AI v/s AI

Feature/Aspect	Generative AI	Traditional AI
Definition	A subset of AI that creates new content (text, images, audio, etc.) based on learned patterns.	AI designed to perform specific tasks by learning from data but typically does not generate new content.
Primary Function	Content creation and synthesis.	Task-specific applications such as classification, prediction, and automation.
Data Input	Uses large datasets to learn patterns for generating new, similar data.	Uses large datasets to learn to perform specific tasks or make decisions.
Output	Generates new, original content like text, images, or music.	Outputs decisions, classifications, predictions, or actions based on input data.

Training Approach	Often employs unsupervised or self-supervised learning, though supervised learning is also common.	Primarily uses supervised learning, reinforcement learning, and sometimes unsupervised learning.
Limitations	Risk of generating biased or inappropriate content; requires large datasets for training.	Limited to predefined tasks; less flexible in adapting to new types of problems.
Interactivity	Can interact with users by generating responses or content based on prompts (e.g., chatbots).	Typically interacts with users by providing results or recommendations based on analysis (e.g., predictive models).

3.3 Edge AI

Edge AI involves executing AI algorithms directly on edge devices, such as smartphones, IoT devices, and autonomous vehicles, rather than depending on cloud-based processing. This local processing ability allows devices to make decisions in milliseconds, without needing an internet connection or cloud access. As the device generates data, the on-board algorithms can immediately utilize this data. Imagine a smart security camera installed in your home. This camera is equipped with Edge AI, allowing it to process video footage locally on the device itself. As it records, the AI algorithms analyse the video in real-time to detect unusual activities or recognize familiar faces. Because the processing happens on the device, the camera can send instant alerts about suspicious movements or unfamiliar faces without needing to upload the footage to the cloud. This ensures not only faster response times but also enhanced privacy and security, as the video data doesn't need to be transmitted over the internet.

With edge AI, machine learning algorithms operate directly at the edge of a network, close to where data is generated, such as on IoT devices or machines equipped with edge computing capabilities. Edge AI devices use embedded algorithms to monitor behaviour, collect, and process data, allowing them to make decisions, automatically correct issues, and predict future performance. Edge AI can run on a variety of hardware, from standard central processing units (CPUs) to microcontrollers and advanced neural processing units. Edge AI is becoming increasingly popular as industries find new ways to leverage its power to optimize workflows, automate business processes, and unlock new opportunities for innovation. This approach also addresses concerns such as latency, security, and cost reduction.

3.4 Quantum AI

Quantum AI is an emerging field that merges the principles of quantum computing with artificial intelligence algorithms to address complex problems that classical computers cannot solve. This combination leverages the power of quantum computing to enable more powerful and efficient AI algorithms, holding significant promise for revolutionizing various industries such as healthcare, finance, and transportation. These advancements could provide solutions that were previously considered impossible. The significance of Quantum AI in advancing AI cannot be overstated. Traditional AI algorithms are constrained by the binary logic and bit-based operations of classical computers. In contrast, Quantum AI utilizes quantum mechanics and quantum computing principles to perform computations with quantum bits, or qubits. This capability allows for the simultaneous exploration of multiple possibilities, potentially leading to exponential speedups in solving certain types of problems.

3.4.3 Potential of Quantum AI

The potential of Quantum AI is vast and can have a significant impact on various industries:

a) Healthcare: Quantum AI can be used to analyse large amounts of medical data and identify patterns that can help in the diagnosis and treatment of diseases. It can also be used to optimize drug discovery processes by simulating the behaviour of molecules and predicting their interactions with target proteins.

b) Finance: Quantum AI can be used to optimize investment portfolios by considering multiple variables simultaneously and identifying the most profitable investment strategies. It can also be used to improve risk management processes by simulating various scenarios and predicting their outcomes.

c) Transportation: Quantum AI can be used to optimize traffic flow and reduce congestion by considering multiple variables, such as traffic volume and road conditions, simultaneously. It can also be used to improve logistics processes by optimizing routes and schedules for delivery vehicles.

d) Supply Chain Optimization: Optimizing delivery chains involves fixing complex logistics and useful resource allocation issues. Quantum Machine Learning should beautify those optimization duties, leading to more efficient aid allocation, decreased prices, and advanced ordinary delivery chain performance.

e) Climate Modelling and Environmental Impact: Quantum computer systems can simulate complex climate fashions greater accurately, enabling higher predictions of weather change consequences and helping inside the development of sustainable regulations to mitigate environmental effect.

f) Cryptography and Security: Quantum computer systems have the potential to break conventional cryptographic systems through algorithms like Shor's set of rules, which could factor large numbers efficiently.

Chapter
04

AI WORKFLOW

Understanding the AI workflow is akin to unravelling the blueprint behind the magic of artificial intelligence. Each stage, meticulously crafted, contributes to the foundation upon which intelligent systems are built. From the initial gathering of data to the final deployment of trained models, every step holds significance in shaping the efficacy and reliability of AI-driven solutions.

4.1 Different Stages of AI Workflow

The AI workflow is characterized by distinct stages, each pivotal in extracting valuable insights from data and converting them into actionable intelligence. Understanding these stages is essential for maximizing the effectiveness of AI applications across domain. Listed below are the different stages.

4.1.1 Data Collection

Data collection is the process of gathering relevant and representative data that the AI model will learn from. The quality and quantity of the data are crucial for the performance of the model.

Process:

1. Identify the types of data needed for the specific AI task (e.g., images, text, and numerical data).
2. Gather data from diverse sources, ensuring it reflects real-world scenarios.

3. Verify the accuracy and completeness of the data to prevent biases and errors.

Data can be gathered from various authenticated sources such as data.gov.in, Kaggle, or the UCI dataset repository. For example, a researcher conducting a scientific study meticulously selects the most trustworthy and pertinent information sources to ensure the accuracy and credibility of the study's results. Similarly, using high-quality and precise data simplifies and improves the model's learning process, ultimately leading to state-of-the-art performance during testing. Collecting such data requires a significant investment of capital, time, and resources. Therefore, organizations and researchers must carefully determine the type of data necessary to achieve their goals or complete their research projects effectively.

Data can be in various forms such as numerical, categorical, or time-series data, and can come from various sources such as databases, spreadsheets, or APIs. Machine learning algorithms use data to learn patterns and relationships between input variables and target outputs, which can then be used for prediction or classification tasks. Data is typically divided into two types:

1. Labelled data
2. Unlabelled data

Labelled data includes a label or target variable that the model is trying to predict, whereas unlabelled data does not include a label or target variable. The data used in machine learning is typically numerical or categorical. Numerical data includes values that can be ordered and measured, such as age or income. Categorical data includes values that represent categories, such as gender or type of fruit.

Data can be divided into training and testing sets. The training set is used to train the model, and the testing set is used to evaluate the performance of the model. It is important to ensure that the data is split in a random and representative way. Big Enterprises are spending lots of money just to gather as much certain data as possible.

Example: Why did Facebook acquire WhatsApp by paying a huge price of $19 billion?

The answer is very simple and logical – it is to have access to the users' information that Facebook may not have but WhatsApp will have. This information about their users is of paramount importance to Facebook as it will facilitate the task of improvement in their services.

How do we split data in Machine Learning?

Training Data: The part of data we use to train our model. This is the data that your model actually sees (both input and output) and learns from.

Validation Data: The part of data that is used to do a frequent evaluation of the model, fit on the training dataset along with improving involved hyperparameters (initially set parameters before the model begins learning). This data plays its part when the model is actually training.

Testing Data: Once our model is completely trained, testing data provides an unbiased evaluation. When we feed in the inputs of testing data, our model will predict some values (without seeing actual output). After prediction, we evaluate our model by comparing it with the actual output present in the testing data. This is how we evaluate and see how much our model has learned from the experiences feed in as training data, set at the time of training.

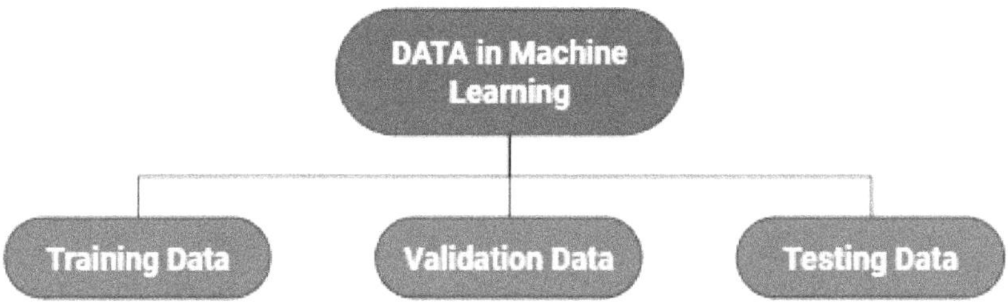

Properties of Data

1. Volume: Scale of Data. With the growing world population and technology at exposure, huge data is being generated each and every millisecond.
2. Variety: Different forms of data – healthcare, images, videos, audio clippings.
3. Velocity: Rate of data streaming and generation.
4. Value: Meaningfulness of data in terms of information that researchers can infer from it.
5. Veracity: Certainty and correctness in data we are working on.
6. Viability: The ability of data to be used and integrated into different systems and processes.
7. Security: The measures taken to protect data from unauthorized access or manipulation.
8. Accessibility: The ease of obtaining and utilizing data for decision-making purposes.
9. Integrity: The accuracy and completeness of data over its entire lifecycle.
10. Usability: The ease of use and interpretability of data for end-users.

Some facts about Data

- With around 5.35 billion internet users worldwide, each person can potentially generate approximately 15.87 TB of data daily.
- Facebook produces approximately 4,000 TB daily, ranking #1 in most visited sites globally in 2023.
- X (Twitter) garners around 500 million tweets daily, which amounts to 560 GB of data.
- In 2024, on average, TikTok videos produce approximately 7.35 TB of data daily.
- YouTube hosted over 720,000 hours of videos daily in 2023, which is equivalent to about 4.3 PB of data.
- Google processes around 3.5 billion searches daily, amounting to 20 PB.

- In 2023, the average internet user created about 1.7 MB of data per second, equal to 146,880 MB daily.
- An average household of 4 can create about 506,736 MB of data daily.

Advantages of using data in Machine Learning

- Improved accuracy: With large amounts of data, machine learning algorithms can learn more complex relationships between inputs and outputs, leading to improved accuracy in predictions and classifications.
- Automation: Machine learning models can automate decision-making processes and can perform repetitive tasks more efficiently and accurately than humans.
- Personalization: With the use of data, machine learning algorithms can personalize experiences for individual users, leading to increased user satisfaction.
- Cost savings: Automation through machine learning can result in cost savings for businesses by reducing the need for manual labour and increasing efficiency.

Disadvantages of using data in Machine Learning

- Bias: Data used for training machine learning models can be biased, leading to biased predictions and classifications.
- Privacy: Collection and storage of data for machine learning can raise privacy concerns and can lead to security risks if the data is not properly secured.
- Quality of data: The quality of data used for training machine learning models is critical to the performance of the model. Poor quality data can lead to inaccurate predictions and classifications.
- Lack of interpretability: Some machine learning models can be complex and difficult to interpret, making it challenging to understand how they are making decisions.

Issues of using data in Machine Learning

- Data quality: One of the biggest issues with using data in machine learning is ensuring that the data is accurate, complete, and representative of the problem domain. Low-quality data can result in inaccurate or biased models.
- Data quantity: In some cases, there may not be enough data available to train an accurate machine learning model. This is especially true for complex problems that require a large amount of data to accurately capture all the relevant patterns and relationships.
- Bias and fairness: Machine learning models can sometimes perpetuate bias and discrimination if the training data is biased or unrepresentative. This can lead to unfair outcomes for certain groups of people, such as minorities or women.
- Overfitting and underfitting: Overfitting occurs when a model is too complex and fits the training data too closely, resulting in poor generalization to new data. Underfitting occurs when a model is too simple and does not capture all the relevant patterns in the data.
- Privacy and security: Machine learning models can sometimes be used to infer sensitive information about individuals or organizations, raising concerns about privacy and security.
- Interpretability: Some machine learning models, such as deep neural networks, can be difficult to interpret and understand, making it challenging to explain the reasoning behind their predictions and decisions.

4.1.2 Data Pre-processing

Data pre-processing involves cleaning and transforming raw data into a format suitable for training the AI model. Data pre-processing is essential for enhancing the quality and reliability of the dataset, ensuring optimal performance during model training and subsequent inference.

Process:

1. Remove or fill missing values in the dataset.
2. Normalize or scale numerical features to a standard range.
3. Encode categorical variables into a numerical format.
4. Split the dataset into training and testing sets for model evaluation.

Remove missing values in the dataset:

This approach is to simply remove rows or columns with missing values from the dataset. This approach is appropriate when the amount of missing data is relatively small and won't significantly affect the analysis. However, if a large portion of the data is missing, removing rows or columns may lead to loss of valuable information and reduced sample size.

Imagine a healthcare dataset with patient records where each row represents a patient and columns represent various attributes like Age, Gender, Blood Pressure, Cholesterol Level, and Diagnosis.

Sample Data (with missing values)

Patient ID	**Age**	**Gender**	**Blood Pressure**	**Cholesterol Level**	**Diagnosis**
1	45	Male	120	180	Hypertension
2	NaN	Female	130	NaN	Diabetes
3	50	Male	NaN	210	Hypertension
4	60	Female	110	NaN	NaN
5	55	NaN	140	200	Heart Disease

Methods for removing Missing Values:

1. Row Removal: Remove entire rows where any column has a missing value.
2. Column Removal: Remove entire columns that have missing values in a significant portion of the data.

Example:

Let's remove rows with any missing values (more aggressive approach):

Patient ID	Age	Gender	Blood Pressure	Cholesterol Level	Diagnosis
1	45	Male	120	180	Hypertension

Only one row remains because rows 2, 3, 4, and 5 have at least one missing value.

Filling Missing Values:

Filling missing values, also known as imputation, refers to the process of handling and substituting missing data points in a dataset. Some of the approaches for filling missing values are as follows:

a. Fill Missing Values with Mean/Median/Mode

Mean/Median/Mode Imputation:

Calculate Means and Modes:

- Age: Mean = (45 + 50 + 60 + 55) / 4 = 52.5
- Blood Pressure: Mean = (120 + 130 + 110 + 140) / 4 = 125
- Cholesterol Level: Mean = (180 + 210 + 200) / 3 = 196.67
- Gender: Mode = Female
- Diagnosis: Mode = Hypertension

Fill missing values

Patient ID	Age	Gender	Blood Pressure	Cholesterol Level	Diagnosis
1	45	Male	120	180	Hypertension
2	52.5	Female	130	196.67	Diabetes
3	50	Male	125	210	Hypertension
4	60	Female	110	196.67	Hypertension
5	55	Female	140	200	Heart Disease

b. Forward Fill

Fill using the previous values in the column.

Patient ID	Age	Gender	Blood Pressure	Cholesterol Level	Diagnosis
1	45	Male	120	180	Hypertension
2	45	Female	130	180	Diabetes
3	50	Male	130	210	Hypertension
4	60	Female	110	210	Hypertension
5	55	Female	140	200	Heart Disease

c. Backward Fill:

Fill using the next values in the column.

Patient ID	Age	Gender	Blood Pressure	Cholesterol Level	Diagnosis
1	45	Male	120	180	Hypertension
2	50	Female	130	210	Diabetes
3	50	Male	110	210	Hypertension
4	60	Female	110	200	Heart Disease
5	55	NaN	140	200	Heart Disease

d. Interpolation:

Use interpolation to estimate the missing values.

Patient ID	Age	Gender	Blood Pressure	Cholesterol Level	Diagnosis
1	45	Male	120	180	Hypertension
2	50	Female	130	195	Diabetes
3	50	Male	125	210	Hypertension
4	60	Female	110	200	Hypertension
5	55	NaN	140	200	Heart Disease

Normalize or scale numerical features to a standard range:

Normalizing or scaling numerical features to a standard range is an essential step in preparing data for many machine learning algorithms. This process ensures that all numerical features contribute equally to the model, preventing features with larger ranges from dominating those with smaller ranges. There are several methods for normalization and scaling, including Min-Max Scaling and Z-score Standardization,

1. Min-Max Scaling

Min-Max Scaling transforms features to a fixed range, usually [0, 1]. This is done by subtracting the minimum value of the feature and then dividing by the range of the feature.

Here's the formula for normalization:

$$X' = \frac{X - X_{min}}{X_{max} - X_{min}}$$

- When X is minimum value, the numerator is zero (Xmin - Xmin) and hence, the normalized value is 0
- When X is maximum value, the numerator is equal to the denominator (Xmax - Xmin) and hence, the normalized value is 1
- When X is neither minimum nor maximum, the normalized value is between 0 and 1. This is referred to as min-max scaling technique

Min-max scaling is a good choice when:

1. The approximate upper and lower bounds of the dataset is known, and the dataset has few or no outliers
2. When the data distribution is unknown or non-Gaussian, and the data is approximately uniformly distributed across the range
3. When maintaining the distribution's original shape is essential

Z-score Standardization (Standard Scaling)

Z-score Standardization transforms features to have a mean of 0 and a standard deviation of 1. This method is useful when the features have different units or scales.

Here's the formula for standardization:

$$X' = \frac{X - \mu}{\sigma}$$

μ is the mean of the feature values and σ is the standard deviation of the feature values. Note that, in this case, the values are not restricted to a particular range.

This technique is particularly useful when dealing with algorithms that assume normally distributed data, such as many linear models. Unlike the min-max scaling technique, feature values are not restricted to a specific range in the standardization technique. This normalization technique basically represents features in terms of the number of standard deviations that lie away from the mean.

Encode categorical variables into a numerical format:

Encoding categorical variables into a numerical format is a common pre-processing step in machine learning and data analysis. There are several methods to achieve this, depending on the nature of the categorical data and the requirements of the machine learning model. Here are the most common methods:

1. Label Encoding: Each unique category is assigned an integer value. This method is suitable when the categorical variable has an intrinsic order (ordinal data).

Example: Severity of a condition (Mild, Moderate, Severe)

Severity	Label Encoded
Mild	0
Moderate	1
Severe	2

Here, the severity levels have a natural order, so label encoding is appropriate.

2. One-Hot Encoding: Each category is converted into a binary vector where only one element is 1 (indicating the presence of the category) and the rest are 0. This method is suitable for nominal data where there is no intrinsic order among categories.

Example: Type of medical insurance (None, Public, Private)

Insurance Type	None	Public	Private
None	1	0	0
Public	0	1	0
Private	0	0	1

This is useful when the categories have no intrinsic order.

3. Ordinal Encoding: Similar to label encoding, but used explicitly for ordinal data where there is a meaningful order among categories.

Example: Stages of cancer (Stage I, Stage II, Stage III, Stage IV)

Cancer Stage	Ordinal Encoded
Stage I	1
Stage II	2
Stage III	3
Stage IV	4

This method respects the natural progression order of cancer stages.

Split the dataset into training and testing sets for model evaluation:

In machine learning data pre-processing, we divide our dataset into a training set and test set. This is one of the crucial steps of data pre-processing as by doing this, we can enhance the performance of our machine learning model.

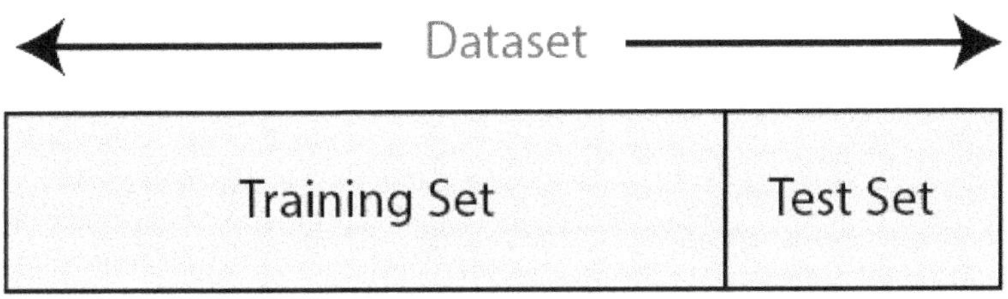

Training Set: A subset of dataset to train the machine learning model, and we already know the output.

Test set: A subset of dataset to test the machine learning model, and by using the test set, model predicts the output.

Advantages of data processing in Machine Learning

1. Improved model performance: Data processing helps improve the performance of the ML model by cleaning and transforming the data into a format that is suitable for modelling.
2. Better representation of the data: Data processing allows the data to be transformed into a format that better represents the underlying relationships and patterns in the data, making it easier for the ML model to learn from the data.
3. Increased accuracy: Data processing helps ensure that the data is accurate, consistent, and free of errors, which can help improve the accuracy of the ML model.

Disadvantages of data processing in Machine Learning

1. Time-consuming: Data processing can be a time-consuming task, especially for large and complex datasets.

2. Error-prone: Data processing can be error-prone, as it involves transforming and cleaning the data, which can result in the loss of important information or the introduction of new errors.
3. Limited understanding of the data: Data processing can lead to a limited understanding of the data, as the transformed data may not be representative of the underlying relationships and patterns in the data.

4.1.3 Feature Extraction

Feature extraction is the process of selecting, transforming, or creating new features from raw data that are relevant and informative for the AI model to learn patterns and make predictions. It involves identifying key characteristics or patterns within the data that can enhance the model's performance.

Process:

1. Identify the raw data features that are most relevant to the task at hand.
2. Apply techniques such as dimensionality reduction to extract and summarise meaningful information from the raw data.
3. Validate extracted features to ensure they capture relevant information and improve the model's performance.
4. Incorporate the extracted features into the dataset for subsequent model training and evaluation

Example: In a medical context, suppose we have a dataset collected from patients to predict the likelihood of developing diabetes.

Identify the raw data features that are most relevant to the task at hand:

The raw data might include:

- Demographic information: age, gender, ethnicity
- Medical history: family history of diabetes, previous diagnoses

- Lifestyle factors: diet, physical activity, smoking status, alcohol consumption
- Clinical measurements: body mass index (BMI), blood pressure, cholesterol levels
- Laboratory tests: fasting blood glucose levels, HbA1c levels, insulin levels

Dimensionality reduction:

Dimensionality reduction techniques like Principal Component Analysis (PCA) can help reduce the number of features while preserving the most important information. Dimensionality reduction is like summarizing all above measurements into a smaller set of key factors or patterns (principal components) that capture most of the important information. It simplifies the dataset without losing important insights.

Suppose you apply dimensionality reduction techniques to the patient dataset. After analysis, you find that you can summarize the complex array of patient measurements into just a few key factors or patterns. For instance:

Factor 1: This factor might capture the overall metabolic health of the patients, incorporating measurements like BMI, fasting blood glucose levels, and HbA1c levels.

Factor 2: This factor could represent cardiovascular health, comprising measurements such as blood pressure and cholesterol levels.

Factor 3: This factor might represent lifestyle factors, including physical activity level and family history of diabetes.

Instead of dealing with each measurement individually, you now have a simplified representation of the data that focuses on the most relevant aspects of the patients' health. This condensed representation not only makes it easier to analyse the data but also helps in identifying overarching patterns and trends that may be crucial for medical diagnosis, risk assessment, or treatment planning.

Validate extracted features:

Validating extracted features is the process of checking to see if the features you've chosen from the raw data are actually helpful for your machine learning model. It's like making sure you picked the right tools for the job. There are two main reasons why this is important:

1. Relevance: You want to make sure the features you're using actually capture information that's related to what you're trying to predict. Imagine training a model to predict house prices, but one of your features is the color of the car parked in the driveway. That feature probably isn't very relevant to the price of the house.
2. Performance: By using relevant features, your model can learn more effectively and make better predictions. Irrelevant features can actually hurt your model's performance by adding noise and complexity.

Here are some common techniques for validating extracted features:

- Correlation analysis: This helps you see how strongly each feature is correlated with the target variable you're trying to predict. Strong correlations suggest the feature might be relevant.
- Feature importance: Some machine learning algorithms can tell you how important each feature was to the model's final predictions. This can help you identify features that weren't very helpful.
- Model performance: Ultimately, the best way to validate features is to see how they affect the model's performance on a held-out test set. If removing a feature improves the model's accuracy, then that feature probably wasn't very helpful.

Incorporate the extracted features into the dataset:

Once you have identified and extracted the most relevant features using techniques like dimensionality reduction, the next step is to integrate these features into your dataset for model training and evaluation. This could involve creating new columns in a data table or constructing a new data matrix where each column represents one of the new features.

Benefits of Feature Incorporation:

- Improved Model Performance: Relevant features often provide more informative data for the model to learn from, leading to better prediction accuracy or classification results.
- Reduced Model Complexity: Dimensionality reduction techniques can help remove redundant or irrelevant information, making the model easier to train and potentially improving its performance.
- Enhanced Interpretability: Some extracted features might be easier to understand than the raw data, aiding in interpreting the model's decisions.

Example: Let's consider a scenario where you're building a machine learning model to predict the risk of heart disease based on patient data. Here's how feature incorporation would play out:

Raw Data Features: You might have raw data like age, gender, blood pressure readings, cholesterol levels, smoking history, etc. These are your base features.

Feature Extraction: You might apply techniques like:

- Feature Engineering: Combine existing features to create a new one, like a Body Mass Index (BMI) calculated from height and weight.
- Dimensionality Reduction: Use Principal Component Analysis (PCA) on blood pressure readings to capture the overall blood pressure trend with fewer features.

Extracted Features: After processing, you might have features like:

- Age
- Gender
- BMI

- Average Blood Pressure (from PCA)
- Smoking Status (Yes/No)

Incorporating Features:

- Add new columns to your dataset for BMI and Average Blood Pressure.
- Calculate the BMI for each patient using height and weight data.
- Assign values for Average Blood Pressure based on the PCA results.

4.1.4 Model Training

Model training is the phase where the AI algorithm learns patterns and relationships from the prepared dataset. During training, the model's parameters are adjusted to minimize the difference between its predictions and the actual labels.

Process:

1. Select an appropriate machine learning or deep learning algorithm based on the task.
2. Feed the training data into the algorithm, allowing it to adjust its internal parameters.
3. Use an optimization algorithm to iteratively refine the model's parameters.
4. Monitor the model's performance on a validation set to avoid overfitting and underfiiting

Algorithm Selection:

Selecting the right algorithm is a crucial step in the model training process. This choice significantly impacts the model's performance, training time, and complexity. The selection process involves understanding the problem type, the nature of the data, computational resources required etc.

Problem Types:

1. Classification: This involves predicting a discrete category, like "spam" or "not spam" in an email filter.

   Common algorithms: Logistic Regression, Support Vector Machines (SVM), K-Nearest Neighbors (KNN), Random Forest, Decision Trees, and Deep Neural Networks (DNNs)

2. Regression: This involves predicting a continuous value, like predicting house prices or stock prices.

   Common algorithms: Linear Regression, Polynomial Regression, Support Vector Regression (SVR), Random Forest Regression, and DNNs

3. Clustering: This involves grouping similar data points together without any pre-defined labels.

   Common algorithms: K-Means clustering, Hierarchical clustering, and DBSCAN

The nature of the data: The characteristics of the dataset influence algorithm selection:

- Data Size: Some algorithms scale better with large datasets (e.g., neural networks) while others perform well on smaller datasets (e.g., decision trees).
- Dimensionality: High-dimensional data might require algorithms that can handle feature selection or dimensionality reduction (e.g., Support Vector Machines, Principal Component Analysis).
- Data Type: The type of data (e.g., numerical, categorical, text, images) determines suitable algorithms. For instance:
  - Text Data: Natural Language Processing (NLP) algorithms, such as RNNs or Transformers.
  - Image Data: Convolutional Neural Networks (CNNs).
  - Tabular Data: Decision Trees, Random Forests, Gradient Boosting Machines.

Computational resources:

The available computational resources (e.g., CPU, GPU, memory) can limit or expand the choice of algorithms:

- Simple Algorithms: Algorithms like Linear Regression, Logistic Regression, or Naive Bayes require less computational power and can run efficiently on a standard CPU.
- Complex Algorithms: Deep learning models, such as CNNs, RNNs, and Transformers, typically require substantial computational power, often utilizing GPUs or TPUs.

Adjust its internal parameters:

The core objective of feeding data into a machine learning or deep learning algorithm is to allow it to learn from the data by adjusting its internal parameters. This process involves several steps where the algorithm iteratively refines its parameters to minimize the error between its predictions and the actual outcomes.

1. Model Parameters:

- Weights and Biases: In algorithms like neural networks, the primary internal parameters are weights and biases. Weights determine the strength of connections between neurons, while biases adjust the output along with the weighted sum of inputs.
- Coefficients: In linear models like linear regression and logistic regression, coefficients represent the relationship between each feature and the target variable.
- Tree Structures: In decision trees and ensemble methods like Random Forests, the structure of the tree, including the split points and nodes, serves as the internal parameters.

2. Hyperparameters vs. Parameters:

- Hyperparameters: These are settings configured before the training process begins, such as learning rate, number of layers in a neural network, or the number of trees in a Random Forest.

- Parameters: These are the values that the model learns during the training process, such as weights in neural networks or split points in decision trees.

Understanding Optimization Algorithms:

1. Objective Function

- Loss Function: The optimization process starts with defining a loss function (or cost function), which quantifies the error between the model's predictions and the actual labels. Common loss functions include Mean Squared Error (MSE) for regression tasks and Cross-Entropy Loss for classification tasks.
- Goal: The primary goal of the optimization algorithm is to minimize this loss function by adjusting the model's parameters.

2. Gradient Descent

- Basic Concept: Gradient Descent is the most common optimization algorithm used in training machine learning models. It works by calculating the gradient (partial derivative) of the loss function with respect to each parameter, which indicates the direction and rate at which the parameters should be updated to reduce the loss.
- Update Rule: The parameters are updated iteratively by moving in the direction opposite to the gradient. The size of the steps taken is determined by the learning rate, a crucial hyperparameter. The learning rate controls how big the steps are during each iteration. If the learning rate is too high, the model might overshoot the minimum; if it's too low, the model will converge very slowly.

3. Variants of Gradient Descent

- Batch Gradient Descent: Uses the entire dataset to compute the gradient of the loss function. This approach ensures a stable convergence but can be computationally expensive and slow for large datasets.

- Stochastic Gradient Descent (SGD): Updates the model parameters using the gradient computed from a single randomly selected data point. This approach is much faster but introduces more noise into the gradient updates, which can sometimes help in escaping local minima.
- Mini-Batch Gradient Descent: A compromise between batch gradient descent and SGD, this approach updates the parameters using the gradient computed from a small random subset of the dataset (mini-batch). It balances the computational efficiency and the stability of the gradient updates.

4. Advanced Optimization Algorithms

- Momentum: Enhances the gradient descent by adding a fraction of the previous update to the current update, helping to accelerate convergence and navigate through valleys.
- RMSprop: Adapts the learning rate for each parameter by dividing the gradient by an exponentially decaying average of past squared gradients, which helps to deal with the problem of vanishing learning rates.
- Adam (Adaptive Moment Estimation): Combines the ideas of momentum and RMSprop. It computes adaptive learning rates for each parameter and maintains running averages of both the gradients and their squares. Adam is widely used due to its efficiency and good performance in practice.

Model Performance monitoring

Monitoring the model's performance on a validation set is a crucial step in the model training process. It helps ensure that the model generalizes well to new, unseen data and avoids the pitfalls of overfitting and underfitting.

1. Definition and Purpose:

- Validation Set: A subset of the dataset that is not used in the training process but is used to evaluate the model's performance.

Typically, the data is split into training, validation, and test sets. The validation set helps tune the model and make decisions about hyperparameters and model architecture.

- Purpose: The primary purpose of the validation set is to provide an unbiased evaluation of the model during training. It helps in detecting overfitting and underfitting by comparing the model's performance on training data and validation data.

Data Splitting:

- Holdout Method: The dataset is randomly split into training and validation sets, often using a ratio such as 80/20 or 70/30.
- Cross-Validation: For a more robust evaluation, techniques like k-fold cross-validation can be used. The data is split into k subsets, and the model is trained k times, each time using a different subset as the validation set and the remaining subsets as the training set. The results are averaged to provide a more reliable performance estimate.

Overfitting and Underfitting

1. Overfitting:

- Definition: Overfitting occurs when the model learns the training data too well, capturing noise and outliers, leading to poor generalization to new data.
- Detection: A model that performs exceptionally well on the training set but poorly on the validation set is likely overfitting. Large gaps between training and validation performance metrics indicate overfitting.

Prevention Techniques:

- Regularization: Techniques like L1 and L2 regularization add a penalty to the loss function for large coefficients, discouraging overly complex models.

- Dropout: In neural networks, randomly dropping units (along with their connections) during training helps prevent overfitting by encouraging the model to learn more robust features.
- Early Stopping: Monitoring validation performance and stopping training when the performance no longer improves (or starts to degrade) helps prevent overfitting.

Underfitting:

- Definition: Underfitting occurs when the model is too simple to capture the underlying patterns in the data, leading to poor performance on both the training and validation sets.
- Detection: A model that performs poorly on both the training and validation sets is likely underfitting. This indicates that the model has not learned enough from the data.

Prevention Techniques:

- Model Complexity: Increasing the complexity of the model by adding more features, layers, or using a more complex algorithm can help.
- Feature Engineering: Creating new features or selecting more relevant features can improve the model's ability to capture underlying patterns.
- Longer Training: Sometimes, simply training the model for more epochs or iterations allows it to learn more effectively.

4.1.5 Evaluation

Model evaluation assesses how well the trained AI model generalizes to new, unseen data. It helps measure the model's performance and identify areas for improvement.

Process:

1. Use a separate dataset (testing set) not seen by the model during training for evaluation.

2. Calculate relevant metrics such as accuracy, precision, recall, or F1 score depending on the task.
3. Analyse the model's performance and identify any issues like overfitting or underfitting.
4. Iterate and fine-tune the model based on evaluation results

Separate test data:

One of the most crucial steps in the process of model evaluation is the use of a separate dataset, known as the testing set, which the model has not encountered during its training phase. This step is essential for several reasons:

1. Ensuring Generalization

The primary goal of training a machine learning model is to enable it to generalize well to new, unseen data. Generalization refers to the model's ability to perform accurately on data that was not part of its training. By evaluating the model on a testing set that it has not seen before, we get an unbiased estimate of how well the model will perform in real-world scenarios where the data is new and potentially different from the training data.

2. Preventing Overfitting

Overfitting occurs when a model learns the training data too well, including its noise and outliers, to the detriment of its performance on new data. This often happens when a model is excessively complex relative to the amount and variability of the training data. Using a testing set helps in identifying overfitting. If the model performs significantly better on the training set than on the testing set, it indicates that the model might be overfitted.

3. Providing an Objective Evaluation

The testing set serves as an objective means to evaluate the model's performance. Since the model has no prior exposure to the testing data, its performance on this data provides a clear and unbiased picture of its effectiveness. This objectivity is crucial for assessing the true predictive power of the model and ensuring that the results are not skewed by any biases present in the training data.

Performance metrics

Once the model has been trained and evaluated using a separate testing set, the next critical step in model evaluation is the calculation of relevant performance metrics. These metrics help quantify how well the model is performing in terms of accuracy, precision, recall, F1 score, and other task-specific measures. The choice of metrics depends on the nature of the problem the model is designed to solve.

Common Metrics

1. Accuracy:

- ❖ Definition: Accuracy is the proportion of correctly predicted instances out of the total instances.
- ❖ Use Case: Accuracy is a suitable metric for balanced datasets where the number of instances in each class is roughly equal.
- ❖ Formula: Accuracy = $\frac{\text{Number of correct prediction}}{\text{Total number of predictions}}$

Accuracy can be represented as $\frac{\mathbf{TP+TN}}{\mathbf{TP+TN+FP+FN}}$

Where, True positive (TP): predicted to be positive and the actual value is also positive
False positive (FP): predicted to be positive but the actual value is negative
True negative (TN): predicted to be negative and the actual value is also negative
False negative (FN): predicted to be negative but the actual value is positive

2. Precision:

- ❖ Definition: Precision is the proportion of true positive predictions out of all positive predictions made by the model.
- ❖ Use Case: Precision is crucial in scenarios where the cost of false positives is high, such as in spam detection or medical diagnostics.
- ❖ Formula: Precision $= \frac{TP}{TP + FP}$

3. Recall (Sensitivity or True Positive Rate):

- ❖ Definition: Recall is the proportion of true positive predictions out of all actual positive instances.
- ❖ Use Case: Recall is important when the cost of false negatives is high, such as in disease screening or fraud detection.
- ❖ Formula: Recall $= \frac{TP}{TP + FN}$

4. F1 Score:

- ❖ Definition: The F1 score is the harmonic mean of precision and recall, providing a single metric that balances both concerns.
- ❖ Use Case: The F1 score is useful when there is an uneven class distribution or when both false positives and false negatives are important.
- ❖ Formula: F1 Score $= 2\times \frac{Precision \times Recall}{Precision + Recall}$

Choosing the Right Metric

The selection of appropriate metrics is dictated by the specific requirements and constraints of the task:

- Binary Classification: Metrics such as accuracy, precision, recall, F1 score, and AUC-ROC are typically used.
- Multiclass Classification: Accuracy, macro-averaged F1 score, and confusion matrices help in understanding performance across multiple classes.

- Regression: MAE, MSE, Root Mean Squared Error (RMSE), and R-squared are standard metrics.
- Imbalanced Datasets: Precision, recall, and the F1 score are preferred over accuracy to provide a more nuanced evaluation.

Interpreting Metrics

- Accuracy: High accuracy indicates a high number of correct predictions but may be misleading if the dataset is imbalanced.
- Precision and Recall: High precision indicates fewer false positives, while high recall indicates fewer false negatives. Depending on the application, one may be prioritized over the other.
- F1 Score: A high F1 score indicates a good balance between precision and recall, making it a comprehensive metric in many contexts.

4.1.6 Deployment

Deployment involves implementing the trained model for real-world use. This step allows the model to make predictions or perform tasks on new, incoming data.

Process:

1. Integrate the model into the target system or application.
2. Set up appropriate infrastructure to support the model's deployment (e.g., server, cloud environment).
3. Implement APIs or interfaces for communication between the model and other components.
4. Monitor the model's performance in a production environment.

Integrating the Model into the Target System or Application:

Integrating the trained machine learning model into the target system or application is the first crucial step in deployment. This essentially bridges the gap between the development environment where the model was built and the real-world scenario where it will be used. Here's a breakdown of what this integration might involve:

- Data Pipeline Development:

  Establish a seamless flow of data from the source (where new data is generated) to the deployed model. This might involve building scripts or connectors to extract and format data for the model's consumption.

- Model Packaging:

  Prepare the model for deployment. This could involve converting it into a format compatible with the target system's programming language or environment. Tools like TensorFlow Serving or ONNX Runtime can be used for this purpose.

- Model Serving Logic:

  Develop code that handles incoming requests, feeds data to the model, and returns the model's predictions or outputs. This code essentially acts as an interface between the application and the model.

- Error Handling:

  Implement mechanisms to handle potential errors during model execution. This might involve checks for invalid data formats, unexpected inputs, or model failures.

- Version Control:

  Establish a version control system for the deployed model. This allows for tracking changes, rolling back to previous versions if needed, and simplifies future updates.

Set up appropriate infrastructure:

Setting up the appropriate infrastructure is crucial for the successful deployment of a machine learning model. This infrastructure ensures that the model can handle real-world data, scale as needed, and remain available and responsive. The process involves several key considerations and steps:

1. Choose the Deployment Environment

Decide whether the model will be deployed on-premises, in the cloud, or in a hybrid setup. Each option has its own advantages and trade-offs:

- On-premises: Offers full control over hardware and data but may require significant upfront investment in infrastructure and maintenance.
- Cloud: Provides scalability, flexibility, and reduced maintenance costs. Popular cloud providers include AWS, Google Cloud Platform (GCP), and Microsoft Azure.
- Hybrid: Combines the benefits of both on-premises and cloud deployments, allowing sensitive data to be kept on-premises while leveraging cloud resources for scalability.

2. Choosing Infrastructure

- Model Requirements: The chosen infrastructure should have the processing power, memory, and storage capacity to handle the model's computational needs.
- Scalability: The environment should be easily scalable to accommodate increased traffic or changing model demands.
- Cost: Cloud platforms offer pay-as-you-go models, while on-premise servers require upfront hardware investments.
- Security: The environment needs robust security measures to protect sensitive data and prevent unauthorized access to the model.

3. Additional Infrastructure Considerations

- Databases: If the model requires persistent storage for training data or intermediate results, a reliable database solution needs to be integrated.

- Monitoring Tools: Monitoring tools should be implemented to track model performance, resource utilization, and potential errors in real-time.
- Load Balancing: For high traffic scenarios, load balancers can distribute requests across multiple instances of the model, ensuring consistent performance.

Relevance of APIs

Imagine your trained model is a new specialist in your hospital. Creating clear communication channels between this specialist and the rest of the medical staff is essential. Here's how it works:

- APIs (Application Programming Interfaces) act as translators. They take information from the patient's medical records (electronic health record system) and translate it into a format the model understands. Similarly, the API translates the model's insights (predictions) back into a way that's clear for doctors and nurses to interpret.
- Think of it like a common language. Just like you wouldn't expect a cardiologist to understand a radiologist's report without some explanation, the API ensures everyone involved can understand each other.
- This clear communication is crucial. It allows doctors to seamlessly incorporate the model's insights into their decision-making process, ultimately improving patient care.

4.1.7 Feedback Loop

The feedback loop is a continuous process of improving the AI model based on new data and user feedback. It helps adapt the model to changing conditions and enhance its performance over time.

Process:

1. Collect feedback from users or system logs to identify areas for improvement.
2. Update the model periodically with new data to keep it current and relevant.
3. Monitor for changes in the data distribution that may impact model performance.
4. Iteratively refine the model based on feedback and evolving requirements.

4.2 Example of AI Workflow: Predicting the developing of diabetes

Let's take an example from the medical sector where we aim to develop an AI model to predict the likelihood of patients developing diabetes based on various health parameters. Here's how each stage of the AI workflow would be implemented:

1. Data Collection

Data collection involves gathering relevant medical data from various sources such as electronic health records (EHRs), patient surveys, lab test results, and wearable health devices.

- Data Sources: Hospitals, clinics, diagnostic labs, and wearable devices.
- Data Types: Patient demographics (age, gender), medical history, blood glucose levels, BMI, blood pressure, cholesterol levels, lifestyle factors (diet, exercise), and family history of diabetes.

2. Data Pre-processing

Pre-processing ensures that the collected data is clean, consistent, and suitable for training the AI model.

- Cleaning: Handling missing values (e.g., imputing missing blood glucose levels), removing duplicates, and correcting errors.

- Normalization: Scaling features like blood glucose levels, BMI, and cholesterol to a standard range.
- Encoding: Converting categorical variables (e.g., gender, lifestyle factors) into numerical values using techniques like one-hot encoding.
- Splitting: Dividing the dataset into training, validation, and test sets.

3. Model Training

Training the AI model involves using the pre-processed data to train a machine learning algorithm to recognize patterns and make predictions.

- Algorithm Selection: Choosing an appropriate algorithm (e.g., logistic regression, decision trees, neural networks).
- Training Process: Feeding the training data into the algorithm and adjusting parameters to minimize prediction error.
- Hyperparameter Tuning: Optimizing the model's hyperparameters (e.g., learning rate, number of layers in a neural network) to improve performance.

4. Evaluation

Evaluating the trained model to assess its performance and ensure it can make accurate predictions on new, unseen data.

- Metrics: Using evaluation metrics such as accuracy, precision, recall, F1 score, and AUC-ROC curve to measure the model's performance.
- Validation Set: Testing the model on a separate validation set to tune the model further and prevent overfitting.
- Test Set: Final evaluation on the test set to determine the model's generalization capability.

5. Deployment

Deploying the trained and evaluated model into a real-world healthcare setting where it can assist medical professionals.

- Integration: Integrating the model into the hospital's EHR system or a mobile health app.
- Accessibility: Ensuring that the model is easily accessible by healthcare providers and potentially patients.
- Real-time Predictions: Enabling the model to make real-time predictions and provide recommendations during patient visits.

6. Feedback Loop

Implementing a feedback loop to continually monitor and improve the model's performance based on real-world data and outcomes.

- Monitoring: Tracking the model's predictions and comparing them with actual patient outcomes.
- Updating: Retraining the model periodically with new data to improve accuracy and adapt to changes in patient populations.
- User Feedback: Collecting feedback from healthcare providers on the model's usability and effectiveness, and making necessary adjustments.

Chapter 05

CURRENT HEALTHCARE SYSTEM

The current healthcare system is a complex and multifaceted network designed to provide medical care and support to populations. It encompasses various stakeholders, including patients, healthcare providers, administrators, insurers, policymakers, and regulators, each playing a crucial role in the system's functioning. Here's an overview of the key components and challenges of the current healthcare system:

1. Patients and Patient Advocacy Groups: Patients are central to the healthcare system, and their experiences, outcomes, and satisfaction are critical measures of system performance. Patient advocacy groups work to represent patients' interests, provide support, and influence healthcare policies.
2. Healthcare Providers: This group includes doctors, nurses, pharmacists, therapists, and other medical professionals who deliver care directly to patients. They work in various settings, including hospitals, clinics, nursing homes, and private practices.
3. Hospitals and Clinics: These facilities provide a range of services from emergency care to routine check-ups and specialized treatments. Hospitals are often categorized into general, specialty, and teaching hospitals.
4. Healthcare Administrators and Managers: These professionals oversee the operations of healthcare facilities, manage budgets, ensure compliance with regulations, and work to improve the quality and efficiency of care.
5. Academic and Research Institutions: Universities, medical schools, and research institutions conduct vital research that advances

medical knowledge, develops new treatments, and trains the next generation of healthcare professionals.

6. Primary Care: Primary care providers (PCPs) serve as the first point of contact for patients. They manage overall patient health, provide preventive care, and coordinate with specialists as needed.
7. Specialty Care: Specialists focus on specific areas of medicine, such as cardiology, oncology, or orthopedics. They provide advanced treatments and procedures that primary care physicians may not be equipped to handle.
8. Insurance and Payers: Health insurance companies and government programs (like Medicare and Medicaid in the United States, Ayushman Bharat - Pradhan Mantri Jan ArogyaYojana (PM-JAY) in India) help cover the cost of medical care. They negotiate rates with providers, manage claims, and offer various plans to individuals and employers.
9. Pharmaceutical and Medical Device Companies: These companies research, develop, and manufacture drugs, medical devices, and other healthcare products. They play a critical role in advancing medical technology and treatment options.
10. Government and Regulatory Bodies: Governments at various levels regulate healthcare through policies, funding, and oversight. Regulatory bodies ensure the safety and efficacy of medical products and services.
11. Public Health Organizations: These organizations focus on population health, disease prevention, and health promotion. They conduct research, provide education, and implement programs to improve community health.

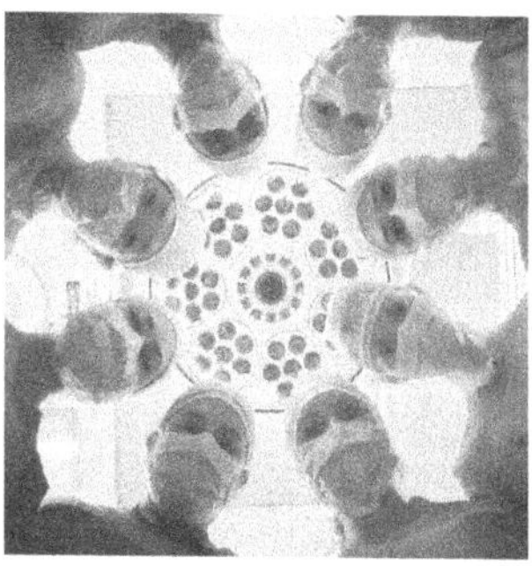

12. Medical and Professional Associations: Organizations like the American Medical Association (AMA), the American Nurses Association (ANA), Indian Medical

Association (IMA), Trained Nurses' Association of India (TNAI) and specialty-specific groups advocate for their members, set professional standards, and provide education and resources.

13. Health Information Technology Companies: These companies develop and provide software and technology solutions that support healthcare delivery, such as electronic health records (EHRs), health information exchanges (HIEs), and telehealth platforms.

5.1 Issues in Current Healthcare System

Despite significant advancements in medical science and technology, the healthcare system continues to face numerous challenges that impact its efficiency, accessibility, and overall effectiveness. These issues are multifaceted, involving economic, social, and technological dimensions, and they vary significantly across different regions and populations.

In the context of exploring the transformative potential of AI in healthcare, it's essential to first understand the existing challenges within the healthcare system. These issues highlight the critical areas where AI technologies can make a significant impact, improving efficiency, accessibility, and patient outcomes.

5.1.1 Access to Healthcare

Access to healthcare involves the ability to obtain services such as preventive care, diagnosis, treatment, and management of health conditions. For healthcare to be considered accessible, it must be both affordable and convenient. However, many individuals, even in developed countries, face challenges in accessing adequate healthcare despite existing government policies and programs. The issue of healthcare inaccessibility is not only a public policy concern but also a moral one. Healthcare professionals, institutions, and governments face controversial choices about providing adequate healthcare like:

a. Resource Allocation

- Prioritizing Treatments: Deciding which treatments and services to prioritize can be controversial, especially when resources are limited. This includes decisions about funding for expensive treatments, elective procedures, and cutting-edge technologies versus more basic, essential care.
- Allocation of Limited Resources: In times of scarcity, such as during pandemics or natural disasters, deciding how to allocate limited resources like ventilators, ICU beds, and vaccines can raise ethical concerns.
- Disparities in Access: Marginalized and rural communities often face significant barriers to receiving medical services, including a lack of healthcare facilities, transportation issues, and shortages of healthcare providers. These disparities result in delayed care, worse health outcomes, and higher mortality rates.

b. Healthcare Rationing

- Age and Quality of Life: Rationing healthcare based on factors such as age, quality of life, or potential for recovery can be highly controversial and raise ethical questions about the value of life and equitable treatment.
- Insurance Coverage: Decisions about what treatments and medications are covered by insurance plans can limit access to care for some individuals, especially those with rare or expensive conditions.

c. Healthcare Funding

- Public vs. Private Funding: The debate over the extent to which healthcare should be publicly funded versus privately funded is ongoing. Public funding may increase accessibility but often requires higher taxes, while private funding can lead to disparities in care based on income.

- Cost-Effectiveness: Determining which treatments and interventions are cost-effective and should be funded can lead to controversial decisions, particularly when expensive treatments offer limited benefits.

d. Health Inequities

- Addressing Social Determinants: Controversy arises in deciding how much responsibility healthcare systems should take for addressing social determinants of health, such as housing, education, and nutrition, which can significantly impact health outcomes.
- Targeted Programs: Implementing targeted health programs for specific populations (e.g., low-income, racial minorities) can be controversial, with debates about fairness and resource allocation.

e. End-of-Life Care

- Assisted Dying and Euthanasia: Legalizing and regulating assisted dying or euthanasia is a highly contentious issue, with strong arguments on both sides regarding patient autonomy, quality of life, and ethical considerations.
- Life-Sustaining Treatments: Decisions about when to withdraw or withhold life-sustaining treatments, such as mechanical ventilation or feeding tubes, can be deeply controversial, involving considerations of patient wishes, family desires, and medical judgment.

f. Medical Research and Innovation

- Experimental Treatments: The use of experimental treatments and participation in clinical trials can raise ethical questions about patient safety, informed consent, and equitable access to new therapies.
- Genetic Editing and Reproductive Technologies: Advances in genetic editing and reproductive technologies (e.g., CRISPR,

IVF) pose ethical dilemmas regarding the extent to which these technologies should be used and regulated.

g. Privacy and Data Security

- Data Sharing: Balancing the benefits of data sharing for medical research and public health against concerns about patient privacy and data security can be contentious.
- Consent and Control: Ensuring that patients have control over their health data and understand how it is used can be challenging, especially with the increasing digitization of health records.

5.1.2 Limited Doctor-Patient Interaction

The doctor-patient relationship lies at the heart of effective healthcare delivery, and the time spent between a doctor and patient is invaluable. This interaction is not merely a formality but a crucial aspect of providing high-quality care, fostering trust, improving patient satisfaction, and ultimately enhancing health outcomes. However, doctors often struggle to allocate sufficient time for patient consultations due to various challenges within the healthcare system.

Importance of Doctor-Patient Interaction

- Building Trust and Rapport: Spending time with patients allows doctors to establish trust and rapport, creating a supportive environment where patients feel comfortable discussing their concerns, symptoms, and treatment preferences openly.
- Gaining Insights into Patient's Health: In-depth conversations enable doctors to gain a comprehensive understanding of the patient's medical history, lifestyle factors, and social determinants of health, and psychosocial context, which are essential for accurate diagnosis and personalized treatment planning.
- Educating and Empowering Patients: Meaningful interactions empower patients with knowledge about their health conditions, treatment options, and self-management strategies, enabling

them to actively participate in decision-making and adhere to treatment plans.

- Addressing Emotional and Psychological Needs: Patients often experience anxiety, fear, or uncertainty about their health, which can impact their well-being and treatment outcomes. Spending time with patients allows doctors to address their emotional and psychological needs, providing reassurance, empathy, and support throughout their healthcare journey.
- Preventing Medical Errors and Adverse Events: Effective communication between doctors and patients helps clarify medical instructions, treatment plans, and medication regimens, reducing the risk of misunderstandings, medication errors, and adverse events.

Challenges Faced by Doctors

- ➢ Time Constraints: Doctors face immense pressure to see a large number of patients within limited appointment slots, leaving insufficient time for each consultation. According to a survey conducted by the Physicians Foundation in 2020, 8 in 10 physicians reported feeling either overextended or at full capacity, with nearly 70% of physicians spending 10 minutes or less with each patient.
- ➢ Administrative Burden: The administrative burden imposed by documentation requirements, electronic health records (EHR) systems, and insurance-related tasks consumes valuable time that could otherwise be spent with patients. A study published in the Annals of Internal Medicine found that physicians spend nearly two hours on administrative tasks for every hour of direct patient care.
- ➢ Burnout and Workload: High workload, long hours, and burnout among healthcare professionals further exacerbate the challenge of allocating sufficient time for patient interactions. A survey conducted by Medscape in 2021 reported that 42% of physicians

experienced burnout, with time pressures cited as a significant contributing factor.

- Financial Pressures: Fee-for-service reimbursement models incentivize rapid patient turnover, leading to shorter appointment times and reduced opportunities for meaningful doctor-patient interactions. Value-based care models that prioritize quality over quantity may offer potential solutions but require systemic changes and investment in care coordination and support services.

5.1.3 Quality of Care

There are significant disparities in the quality of care across different populations. Problems like misdiagnosis, medical errors, and uneven care contribute to suboptimal health outcomes. According to WHO Quality of care is the degree to which health services for individuals and populations increase the likelihood of desired health outcomes. It is based on evidence-based professional knowledge and is critical for achieving universal health coverage. As nations strive for Health for all, it is essential to focus on both the quality of care and health services.

Key Components of Quality of Care

- Safety: Ensuring that the care provided does not harm patients. This includes minimizing medical errors, preventing infections, and ensuring safe practices in all healthcare settings.
- Effectiveness: Providing services based on scientific knowledge to all who could benefit, and refraining from providing services to those not likely to benefit (i.e., avoiding overuse and underuse of medical interventions).
- Patient-Centeredness: Respecting and responding to individual patient preferences, needs, and values, ensuring that patient values guide all clinical decisions.
- Timeliness: Reducing waiting time and harmful delays for both those who receive and those who provide care.

- Efficiency: Minimizing waste, including the inefficient use of equipment, supplies, ideas, and energyTop of FEquitability: Delivering care that remains consistent in quality regardless of personal factors such as gender, ethnicity, geographic location, or socioeconomic status.

Challenges in Ensuring Quality of Care

- Variation in Care: There is considerable variability in the quality of care provided by different healthcare providers and institutions. This can be due to differences in resources, training, and adherence to evidence-based guidelines.
- Medical Errors: Preventable medical errors are a significant issue, contributing to patient harm and increased healthcare costs. Errors can occur in diagnosis, treatment, and medication administration.
- Access and Equity: Disparities in healthcare access and quality affect marginalized and vulnerable populations disproportionately. Factors such as race, ethnicity, income, and geographic location can influence the quality of care received.
- Patient Engagement: Involving patients in their care is essential for achieving high-quality outcomes. However, there are barriers to effective patient engagement, including health literacy, cultural differences, and communication gaps.
- Continuity of Care: Fragmentation of care, where patients receive services from multiple providers without proper coordination, can lead to gaps in care, repeated tests, and inconsistent treatment plans.
- Health Information Technology: While electronic health records (EHRs) and other health IT systems have the potential to improve quality, issues with interoperability, usability, and data accuracy can hinder their effectiveness.

5.1.4 Healthcare Workforce Shortages

The healthcare workforce is the backbone of any health system, providing essential services that save lives and promote well-being. However, healthcare systems worldwide are facing significant workforce shortages that threaten the quality, accessibility, and sustainability of care. This issue is multifaceted, driven by a range of factors including aging populations, increasing demand for healthcare services, and insufficient training and recruitment of new healthcare professionals.

Key Drivers of Healthcare Workforce Shortages

- Aging Population and Workforce: As population age, the demand for healthcare services rises. Concurrently, many healthcare workers are reaching retirement age, leading to a decrease in the active workforce. This dual challenge exacerbates the strain on healthcare systems, particularly in developed countries.
- Increasing Healthcare Demand: Advancements in medical technology and treatment options have increased the scope and complexity of healthcare services. Additionally, the prevalence of chronic diseases such as diabetes, heart disease, and cancer has surged, necessitating more prolonged and intensive care.
- Training and Education Gaps: There is a significant lag in the number of new healthcare professionals being trained and entering the workforce. Educational institutions face challenges such as limited faculty, insufficient funding, and outdated curricula that do not match current healthcare needs.
- Geographic and Specialty Maldistribution: Even within countries with a relatively adequate overall number of healthcare workers, there is often a maldistribution problem. Rural and underserved urban areas frequently experience severe shortages. Certain specialties, such as primary care, geriatrics, and mental health, also suffer from a lack of professionals.
- Burnout and Job Satisfaction: High levels of stress, burnout, and dissatisfaction are prevalent among healthcare workers due to long

hours, high patient loads, and administrative burdens. This leads to higher turnover rates and deters new entrants to the profession.

Impacts of Healthcare Workforce Shortages

- Reduced Access to Care: Workforce shortages can lead to longer wait times for appointments, delays in treatment, and limited availability of services, particularly in rural and underserved areas.
- Lower Quality of Care: Overburdened healthcare workers may struggle to provide the high-quality care that patients need, potentially leading to medical errors, decreased patient satisfaction, and poorer health outcomes.
- Increased Healthcare Costs: Shortages can drive up healthcare costs due to the need for overtime pay, the hiring of temporary staff, and the inefficiencies associated with an overstretched workforce.
- Public Health Risks: Inadequate healthcare staffing can hinder responses to public health emergencies, such as infectious disease outbreaks or natural disasters, compromising the health and safety of populations.

5.1.5 Updated Discipline V/S Outdated Practitioners

In the dynamic and ever-evolving landscape of healthcare, the clash between updated discipline and outdated practitioners highlights a crucial divide that significantly impacts patient care, outcomes, and the overall quality of healthcare delivery. While many healthcare professionals embrace continuous learning, innovation, and evidence-based practices, others may find themselves lagging behind due to various factors, leading to outdated practices and beliefs. Understanding the reasons behind this phenomenon, its consequences, and potential remedies is essential for advancing healthcare and ensuring optimal patient outcomes.

Why Practitioners Become Outdated:

- Time Constraints: Healthcare professionals often operate in fast-paced, high-pressure environments where time is a precious commodity. The demands of patient care, administrative tasks, and other responsibilities can leave little time for practitioners to dedicate to ongoing education, training, or professional development.
- Resistance to Change: Some practitioners may resist change, clinging to familiar routines, practices, and beliefs even as new evidence, guidelines, and technologies emerge. This resistance may stem from fear of the unknown, inertia, or scepticism regarding the effectiveness or safety of new approaches.
- Limited Access to Education and Resources: Healthcare professionals operating in resource-constrained environments or underserved areas may face barriers to accessing continuing education, training programs, or updated clinical guidelines. Limited access to relevant resources and professional development opportunities can impede their ability to stay abreast of advancements in their field.
- Comfort Zone: Practitioners may become complacent or comfortable with their existing knowledge and skills, failing to recognize the importance of ongoing learning and self-improvement. This complacency can lead to stagnation, professional inertia, and a reluctance to challenge or update established practices.
- Technological Literacy: Rapid advancements in medical technology, digital health solutions, and information systems require healthcare professionals to possess adequate technological literacy and adaptability. Those lacking in these skills may struggle to integrate new technologies into their practice or leverage data-driven approaches to patient care.

Consequences of Outdated Practices

- Suboptimal Patient Outcomes: Outdated practices may fail to align with current standards of care, evidence-based guidelines, or best practices, resulting in suboptimal patient outcomes, prolonged hospital stays, increased complications, and avoidable adverse events.
- Patient Harm: In some cases, outdated practices can directly contribute to patient harm, including misdiagnosis, medication errors, preventable complications, and healthcare-associated infections. These incidents not only compromise patient safety but also erode trust in the healthcare system and individual practitioners.
- Quality of Care: Outdated practices may undermine the overall quality of care delivered, leading to variations in care, inconsistencies in treatment approaches, and disparities in health outcomes across patient populations. This can exacerbate health inequities and contribute to disparities in access, quality, and outcomes.
- Professional Reputation: Practitioners who fail to keep pace with advancements in their field risk damaging their professional reputation, credibility, and trustworthiness among patients, colleagues, and the broader healthcare community. This may impact referrals, career opportunities, and professional satisfaction.

5.1.6 Healthcare cost: A Matter of Life and Wallet

In the modern healthcare landscape, the relentless escalation of healthcare costs stands as a formidable challenge, exerting pressure on healthcare budgets and erecting barriers to access for individuals and communities worldwide. This persistent upward trend in healthcare expenditures not only threatens the financial sustainability of healthcare systems but also exacerbates health inequities, limiting access to essential care and services for vulnerable populations. Understanding the drivers of rising healthcare costs and their far-reaching implications is essential for developing effective strategies to mitigate this growing crisis.

Factors Contributing to Escalating Costs

- Medical Advancements: While medical advancements have led to improved patient outcomes and enhanced treatment options, they often come at a steep price. Innovative drugs, medical devices, and procedures developed through extensive research and development efforts contribute to escalating healthcare costs, as manufacturers seek to recoup their investments and generate profits.
- Aging Population: As population's age and life expectancy increases, the prevalence of chronic diseases, comorbidities, and age-related conditions rises, driving up healthcare utilization and expenditures. Older adults typically require more frequent healthcare services, medications, and long-term care, placing additional strain on healthcare budgets.
- Technological Innovation: Rapid advancements in medical technology, diagnostic imaging, and treatment modalities have revolutionized healthcare delivery but also come with significant costs. High-tech medical equipment, such as MRI machines, robotic surgery systems, and advanced imaging technologies, require substantial investments in infrastructure, maintenance, and personnel training.
- Administrative Complexity: The administrative complexity of healthcare systems, including billing processes, insurance claims, and regulatory compliance requirements, adds administrative overhead that contribute to healthcare costs. Administrative expenses consume a significant portion of healthcare spending, diverting resources away from direct patient care.
- Profit Motive: When healthcare organizations prioritize profit over patient care, decisions may be driven by financial considerations rather than clinical outcomes or patient well-being. Profit-driven

practices may incentivize unnecessary procedures, overprescribing medications, or prioritizing high-margin services over preventive care.

- Fee-for-Service Model: In fee-for-service payment models, healthcare providers are reimbursed based on the volume of services delivered, incentivizing the provision of more services rather than focusing on value or outcomes. This can lead to overutilization of healthcare services, unnecessary tests and procedures, and inflated healthcare costs.
- Market Competition: Intense competition among healthcare providers and insurers to attract patients and maximize revenue can fuel healthcare costs. Providers may invest in expensive medical technology or facilities to gain a competitive edge, driving up costs for consumers and
- Price Inflation: Pharmaceutical companies, medical device manufacturers, and other healthcare entities may engage in price inflation, charging exorbitant prices for drugs, devices, and services to maximize profits. This can pose financial burdens for patients, payers, and healthcare systems, driving up overall healthcare costs.
- Influence on Prescribing Behaviour: Studies have shown that interactions with pharmaceutical representatives and receipt of gifts or payments from pharmaceutical companies can influence prescribing behaviour among healthcare providers. Doctors may be more likely to prescribe brand-name medications over generic alternatives or recommend newer, more expensive drugs, even when equally effective, due to influence from pharmaceutical marketing. Furthermore, these interactions and incentives can also contribute to overprescription practices, leading to unnecessary medication usage and potential patient harm.

5.1.7 Data Deluge: Challenges of Healthcare Data Overload

In today's healthcare landscape, the exponential expansion of data is transforming the way medical professionals manage and analyse information. This surge encompasses a wide array of sources, including electronic health records (EHRs), medical imaging, genetic data, wearable devices, and patient-reported outcomes. The integration of these diverse data streams promises to revolutionize healthcare by providing a more comprehensive understanding of individual patient needs, population health trends, and treatment efficacy.

However, this abundance of data also presents formidable challenges to healthcare systems worldwide. The sheer volume and complexity of healthcare data strain the capacity of traditional analytical methods to extract actionable insights efficiently. Healthcare providers and researchers face the daunting task of sifting through massive datasets to identify meaningful patterns, correlations, and trends. This process is further complicated by the heterogeneous nature of healthcare data, which often resides in disparate systems and formats, making integration and analysis a formidable undertaking.

In the face of this data deluge, healthcare organizations are grappling with critical questions regarding data governance, interoperability, and privacy. Ensuring the security and integrity of sensitive patient information is paramount, requiring robust data management practices and adherence to regulatory guidelines such as the Health Insurance Portability and Accountability Act (HIPAA) of USA as well as broader data protection regulations like The General Data Protection Regulation (GDPR) of European Union, information Technology Act and proposed Digital Information Security in Healthcare Act (DISHA) in India. The consequences of data overload extend beyond the realm of clinical care to impact medical research and healthcare delivery as a whole. Delayed or inadequate analysis of healthcare data may impede efforts to translate research findings into real-world applications, slowing the pace of medical innovation. Furthermore, the inability to extract actionable insights from the vast trove of available data may hinder efforts to improve healthcare quality, reduce costs, and enhance patient outcomes.

5.1.8 Administrative Burden

Administrative burden in healthcare refers to the time, effort, and resources required for healthcare providers, patients, and administrative staff to comply with various regulatory, documentation, and procedural requirements. These burdens can significantly affect the efficiency of healthcare delivery, patient outcomes, and the overall cost of healthcare services.

Types of Administrative Burden in Healthcare

- Documentation Requirements: This includes the extensive paperwork and electronic records that healthcare providers must maintain for patient care, billing, and compliance purposes. Documentation involves patient histories, treatment plans, insurance claims, and regulatory reporting.
- Regulatory Compliance: Healthcare providers must comply with numerous regulations and standards set by government bodies, accreditation organizations, and insurance companies..
- Prior Authorizations: Before providing certain treatments or medications, healthcare providers often need to obtain approval from insurance companies. This process, known as prior authorization, involves significant time and effort to gather and submit the necessary information and await approval.
- Billing and Coding: Accurate billing and coding for healthcare services are essential for reimbursement from insurance companies. This requires detailed knowledge of coding systems like ICD-10 (International Classification of Diseases) and CPT (Current Procedural Terminology), and extensive time for data entry and error correction.
- Patient Coordination: Coordinating care among different healthcare providers, specialists, and facilities involves considerable administrative work. This includes managing referrals, sharing medical records, and ensuring continuity of care.

Causes of Administrative Burden in Healthcare

- Complexity of Regulations: The healthcare industry is highly regulated, with complex and often overlapping requirements from multiple regulatory bodies. This complexity can be overwhelming and difficult to navigate.
- Fragmented Systems: The use of different electronic health record (EHR) systems and lack of interoperability between them can lead to duplication of effort and increased administrative tasks.
- Insurance Requirements: Different insurance plans have varying requirements for documentation, prior authorizations, and billing, adding to the administrative burden.
- Resource Constraints: Healthcare facilities, especially smaller practices, may lack the resources to effectively manage administrative tasks, leading to increased workload for existing staff.

Impacts of Administrative Burden in Healthcare

- Provider Burnout: Excessive administrative tasks contribute to burnout among healthcare providers. Physicians and nurses spend significant portions of their time on paperwork rather than patient care, leading to job dissatisfaction and decreased quality of care.
- Patient Care: Administrative burdens can delay patient care and reduce the time healthcare providers can spend with patients. This can lead to poorer health outcomes and patient dissatisfaction.
- Healthcare Costs: The resources spent on managing administrative tasks add to the overall cost of healthcare. This includes hiring additional administrative staff, investing in EHR systems, and handling billing and compliance issues.
- Access to Care: Patients may face delays in receiving care due to administrative hurdles like prior authorizations and insurance verifications. This can be particularly challenging for patients with chronic conditions or urgent healthcare needs.

5.1.9 Pharmaceutical Practices

Pharmaceutical practices play a crucial role in ensuring that medications are accessible, affordable, and available to those who need them. However, issues related to drug pricing and the availability of medications present significant challenges. These issues can limit patient access to necessary treatments, disrupt patient care, and impact treatment outcomes. This write-up explores the complexities of drug pricing and the factors influencing the availability of medications, highlighting their implications and potential solutions.

1. Drug Pricing

High Costs and Affordability

The high cost of prescription medications is a significant barrier to healthcare access. Several factors contribute to the high prices of drugs, including:

- Research and Development (R&D) Costs: Developing new medications involves extensive research, clinical trials, and regulatory approval processes, which are costly and time-consuming. Pharmaceutical companies often cite these costs as justification for high drug prices.
- Patent Protections: Patents grant pharmaceutical companies exclusive rights to sell a new drug for a certain period, allowing them to set high prices without competition. While patents incentivize innovation, they can also lead to monopolistic pricing practices.
- Marketing and Sales Expenses: Pharmaceutical companies invest heavily in marketing and sales efforts to promote their drugs to healthcare providers and patients, adding to the overall cost of medications.
- Lack of Price Regulation: In many countriesthere is limited regulation on drug prices, allowing pharmaceutical companies to set prices based on market demand and potential profitability.

Impact on Patient Access

High drug prices can have several adverse effects on patient access to medications:

- Financial Barriers: Patients may struggle to afford their prescribed medications, leading to non-adherence to treatment plans and poorer health outcomes. This is particularly challenging for individuals without adequate insurance coverage.
- Influence on Prescribing Behaviours: Pharmaceutical companies' pricing practices and marketing strategies can influence healthcare providers' prescribing behaviours, sometimes leading to the preference for more expensive medications over equally effective, lower-cost alternatives.
- Health Disparities: High drug prices disproportionately affect vulnerable populations, exacerbating health disparities and limiting access to essential treatments for low-income individuals and communities.

2. Availability of Medications

Drug Shortages

The availability of medications is critical for effective patient care. However, drug shortages can significantly disrupt treatment outcomes. Causes of drug shortages include:

- Manufacturing Issues: Problems in the manufacturing process, such as quality control failures, production delays, and supply chain disruptions, can lead to shortages of essential medications.
- Regulatory Challenges: Regulatory hurdles and delays in approving manufacturing changes or new suppliers can contribute to shortages.
- Market Dynamics: Economic factors, such as low-profit margins for certain drugs, can lead manufacturers to discontinue production, resulting in shortages.

- Global Supply Chain Dependencies: Reliance on global supply chains for raw materials and finished products can make the pharmaceutical industry vulnerable to geopolitical tensions, natural disasters, and pandemics, affecting drug availability.

Impact on Patient Care

Drug shortages can significantly impact patient care and treatment and outcomes:

- Treatment Delays: Shortages of critical medications can lead to treatment delays, adversely affecting patient health and recovery, particularly in emergency and acute care settings.
- Use of Alternatives: Healthcare providers may need to use alternative medications, which may be less effective or have different side effect profiles, potentially compromising patient care.
- Increased Costs: Drug shortages can drive up the prices of available alternatives, increasing the financial burden on patients and healthcare systems.

Chapter 06

AI PANACEA IN HEALTHCARE

In the previous chapter, we discussed the healthcare industry, from diagnostic errors and administrative inefficiencies to the high costs of treatment. As we transition into this chapter, we explore how artificial intelligence emerges as a powerful solution to these pressing issues. By leveraging advanced algorithms, vast data sets, and machine learning capabilities, AI holds the potential to revolutionize healthcare, making it more efficient, accurate, and accessible.

The healthcare industry is on the cusp of a revolution, with artificial intelligence poised to be the transformative force that changes the way we diagnose, treat, and manage diseases. AI's potential as a panacea in healthcare lies in its ability to analyse vast amounts of data, provide personalized treatment plans, and optimize administrative processes, all while reducing costs and improving patient outcomes.

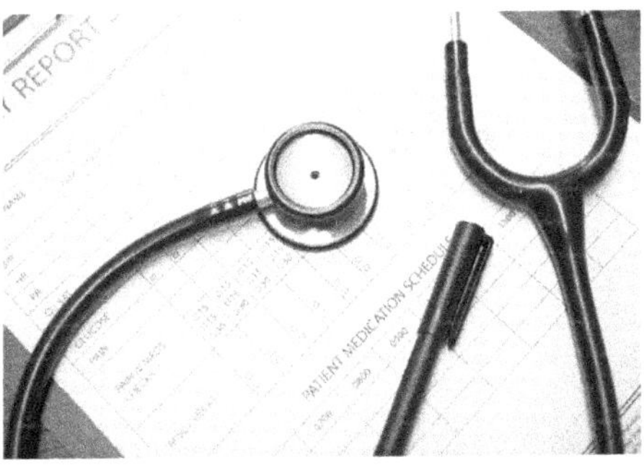

AI can play a transformative role in addressing many of the challenges related to healthcare access and the controversial choices that healthcare professionals, institutions, and governments face. Here's how AI can address each of the specified areas:

6.1 Access to Healthcare

AI plays vital role in mitigating the issue with respect to various aspects of Healthcare accessibility

Prioritizing Treatments

- Predictive Analytics: AI can analyse large datasets to predict which treatments will be most effective for specific populations, helping to prioritize care based on expected outcomes.
- Cost-Benefit Analysis: AI tools can evaluate the cost-effectiveness of various treatments, aiding in decision-making for funding allocations.

Allocation of Limited Resources

- Resource Optimization: AI can optimize the allocation of limited resources during crises by predicting demand and ensuring that supplies such as ventilators and ICU beds are distributed where they are needed most.
- Real-Time Data Analysis: AI systems can analyse real-time data to make dynamic allocation decisions during emergencies, ensuring the most efficient use of resources.

Disparities in Access

- Telemedicine Platforms: AI-driven telemedicine can provide remote consultations to underserved and rural areas, reducing disparities in access to care.
- Outreach and Engagement: AI can identify and engage with marginalized communities to ensure they receive timely and appropriate healthcare services.

Healthcare Rationing

- Ethical Decision-Making Algorithms: AI can incorporate ethical frameworks to support decisions about rationing care based on age, quality of life, and potential recovery outcomes, ensuring more equitable and transparent decision-making.

Insurance Coverage

- Personalized Insurance Plans: AI can help design personalized insurance plans that consider individual health profiles, ensuring better coverage for rare or expensive conditions.
- Claims Management: AI can streamline the claims process, reducing administrative barriers and improving access to necessary treatments.

Healthcare Funding

- Efficiency Improvements: AI can increase the efficiency of healthcare delivery, reducing costs and potentially easing the financial burden on both public and private funding systems.
- Data-Driven Policy Making: AI can provide insights into the impact of different funding models on health outcomes, informing more effective policy decisions.

Cost-Effectiveness

- Treatment Evaluation: AI can assess the cost-effectiveness of treatments and interventions, helping policymakers allocate funds more effectively to maximize health benefits.

Health Inequities

- Comprehensive Data Analysis: AI can analyse data on social determinants of health to identify at-risk populations and develop targeted interventions.
- Predictive Modeling: AI can predict how changes in social determinants (e.g., housing, education) will impact health outcomes, guiding public health initiatives.

Targeted Programs

- Program Evaluation: AI can evaluate the effectiveness of targeted health programs, ensuring resources are used efficiently and equitably.

- Personalized Interventions: AI can design personalized interventions for specific populations, improving health outcomes for low-income and racial minority groups.

End-of-Life Care

Assisted Dying and Euthanasia

- Ethical Decision Support: AI can provide decision support tools that incorporate ethical considerations and patient preferences, aiding in end-of-life care decisions.
- Advanced Directives Management: AI can help manage and respect patients' advanced directives, ensuring their end-of-life wishes are honoured.

Life-Sustaining Treatments

- Prognostic Tools: AI can offer accurate prognostic tools to guide decisions about life-sustaining treatments, helping families and healthcare providers make informed choices.

Medical Research and Innovation

Experimental Treatments

- Clinical Trial Optimization: AI can identify suitable candidates for clinical trials and monitor patient safety, enhancing the ethical conduct of research.
- Informed Consent: AI-driven platforms can ensure patients fully understand the implications of participating in clinical trials, improving informed consent processes.

Genetic Editing and Reproductive Technologies

- Ethical Guidelines Implementation: AI can help implement and monitor adherence to ethical guidelines in the use of genetic editing and reproductive technologies.

- Risk Assessment: AI can assess risks and benefits of new technologies, guiding regulatory decisions.

Privacy and Data Security

Data Sharing

- Secure Data Platforms: AI can develop secure platforms for data sharing that balance the benefits of research with patient privacy protections.
- Anonymization Techniques: AI can anonymize patient data to ensure privacy while enabling valuable medical research.

Consent and Control

- Patient Empowerment Tools: AI can create tools that give patients greater control over their health data, ensuring they understand and consent to its use.
- Data Governance: AI can support robust data governance frameworks, ensuring ethical use of patient information.

By leveraging these AI capabilities, healthcare systems can address many of the challenges associated with access to care, resource allocation, and ethical decision-making, ultimately improving healthcare outcomes and equity.

6.2 Addressing the issue of limited doctor-patient interaction

AI systems play a multifaceted role in addressing the issue of limited doctor-patient interaction and in bolstering trust and rapport between doctors and patients by offering a diverse range of functionalities.

Personalized Communication: AI-powered chatbots and virtual assistants can engage with patients in natural language conversations, providing personalized responses tailored to each individual's needs and preferences. By demonstrating empathy and understanding, these AI systems can help foster a sense of trust and rapport with patients.

Consistent Availability: AI systems operate 24/7, providing consistent availability for patients to seek information, advice, or support whenever they need it. This availability helps build trust by ensuring that patients can access healthcare resources and assistance whenever necessary, without being limited by factors such as office hours or appointment availability.

Evidence-Based Information: AI can provide patients with evidence-based information and recommendations, helping to educate them about their health conditions, treatment options, and preventive measures. By offering reliable and accurate information, AI builds trust by empowering patients to make informed decisions about their health.

Transparent Decision Making: AI-based decision support systems can assist healthcare providers in transparently explaining their decision-making process to patients. By providing insights into the rationale behind treatment recommendations or diagnostic decisions, AI helps patients understand and trust the medical care they receive.

Data Privacy and Security: AI systems can be designed to prioritize patient privacy and security, ensuring that sensitive health information is protected. By implementing robust data protection measures and transparent data handling practices, AI builds trust by demonstrating a commitment to patient confidentiality and confidentiality.

Continuity of Care: AI-powered health monitoring systems can track patients' health metrics continuously, alerting healthcare providers to any concerning changes or trends. By facilitating ongoing monitoring and follow-up care, AI contributes to the continuity of care, helping patients feel supported and cared for over time.

Empathetic Interactions: Advances in natural language processing enable AI systems to recognize and respond to emotional cues in patients' speech or text. By displaying empathy and understanding during interactions, AI helps build rapport with patients, fostering a sense of trust in the healthcare provider's commitment to their well-being.

Feedback and Improvement: AI systems can analyse patient feedback and interactions to continuously improve their performance and responsiveness. By incorporating patient input and preferences into their algorithms, AI systems demonstrate a commitment to patient-centered care, fostering trust and engagement over time.

6.3 Addressing the issue of outdated doctors

AI can play a significant role in mitigating the challenges associated with outdated doctors in several ways:

Continuing Medical Education (CME): AI-powered platforms can provide personalized and up-to-date CME courses tailored to the specific needs and interests of individual doctors. These platforms can utilize machine learning algorithms to track doctors' learning progress, identify areas for improvement, and recommend relevant educational resources accordingly. By keeping doctors abreast of the latest medical advancements and best practices, AI ensures that they maintain competency in their fields despite potential outdated knowledge.

Clinical Decision Support Systems (CDSS): AI-based CDSS can assist outdated doctors in making evidence-based clinical decisions by providing real-time access to the latest medical guidelines, research findings, and treatment protocols. These systems can analyse patient data and medical literature to offer personalized recommendations, helping doctors stay current with evolving standards of care and reducing the risk of outdated practices.

Telemedicine and Remote Consultations: AI-powered telemedicine platforms enable outdated doctors to consult with specialist colleagues or medical experts remotely, regardless of geographical constraints. By facilitating collaborative decision-making and knowledge sharing, these platforms allow doctors to access expertise beyond their own areas of proficiency, ensuring that patients receive the most up-to-date and comprehensive care possible.

Clinical Documentation Assistance: AI-driven clinical documentation tools can assist outdated doctors in accurately documenting patient encounters by automatically generating structured notes, coding diagnoses, and suggesting appropriate treatment plans. By streamlining documentation workflows and reducing the time spent on administrative tasks, these tools enable doctors to focus more on patient care and staying current with medical advancements.

Peer Learning and Collaboration: AI-powered platforms can facilitate peer learning and collaboration among doctors by connecting them with colleagues who have expertise in specific medical areas or recent developments. Through online forums, case discussions, and knowledge-sharing communities, doctors can exchange insights, learn from each other's experiences, and stay updated on emerging trends in healthcare.

6.4 Addressing the issue of Quality of Care

AI can play a crucial role in addressing disparities in the quality of care and ensuring high standards across the key components of quality care. Here's how AI can help:

Key Components of Quality of Care

1. Safety

- Error Reduction: AI can detect potential errors in real-time by analysing patient data, medication orders, and treatment plans, alerting healthcare providers to possible mistakes.
- Infection Prevention: AI-powered systems can monitor hospital environments for infection risks and ensure adherence to hygiene protocols.
- Safe Practices: AI can assist in developing and enforcing standard operating procedures to minimize risks in medical procedures and patient care.

2. Effectiveness

- Evidence-Based Recommendations: AI can provide healthcare providers with the latest evidence-based guidelines and recommendations, ensuring that treatments are up-to-date and effective.
- Outcome Prediction: AI can predict patient outcomes based on historical data and current health status, helping clinicians choose the most beneficial interventions and avoid unnecessary ones.

3. Patient-Centeredness

- Personalized Care: AI can tailor treatment plans to individual patient needs and preferences by analysing data from electronic health records (EHRs) and patient feedback.
- Patient Communication: AI-driven chatbots and virtual assistants can facilitate communication between patients and healthcare providers, addressing questions and concerns in a timely manner.

4. Timeliness

- Appointment Scheduling: AI can optimize scheduling to reduce wait times and ensure patients receive timely care.
- Emergency Response: AI can prioritize cases based on urgency in emergency departments, ensuring that critical patients are attended quickly.

5. Efficiency

- Resource Management: AI can optimize the use of healthcare resources, such as staffing, equipment, and facilities, to avoid waste and improve service delivery.
- Process Automation: AI can automate routine administrative tasks, freeing up healthcare providers to focus more on patient care.

6. Equitability

- Bias Detection: AI can identify and mitigate biases in treatment plans and decision-making processes, ensuring equitable care across diverse populations.
- Access Improvement: AI can analyse data to identify gaps in healthcare access and develop strategies to provide high-quality care to underserved communities.

Challenges in Ensuring Quality of Care

1. Variation in Care

- Standardization: AI can help standardize care by providing guidelines and protocols based on best practices, reducing variability among healthcare providers.
- Training and Education: AI-driven platforms can offer continuous education and training to healthcare providers, ensuring they stay updated with the latest medical knowledge.

2. Medical Errors

- Real-Time Monitoring: AI can continuously monitor patient data for signs of potential errors, such as incorrect medication dosages or conflicting treatments.
- Decision Support: AI-based clinical decision support systems can provide healthcare providers with real-time insights and alerts to prevent errors.

3. Access and Equity

- Telehealth: AI-powered telehealth services can provide high-quality care to remote and underserved populations, reducing disparities in access and quality.
- Outreach Programs: AI can help design and implement targeted outreach programs to improve access to care for marginalized communities.

4. Patient Engagement

- Health Literacy: AI can offer educational resources tailored to different literacy levels and languages, improving patient understanding and engagement.
- Communication Tools: AI-driven communication tools can bridge cultural and language gaps, enhancing patient-provider interactions.

5. Continuity of Care

- Care Coordination: AI can integrate data from multiple providers and ensure seamless communication and coordination, reducing fragmentation and improving continuity.
- Patient Tracking: AI can track patient progress across different healthcare settings, ensuring consistent and continuous care.

6. Health Information Technology

- Interoperability: AI can facilitate the integration and interoperability of EHRs and other health IT systems, ensuring smooth data flow and accessibility.
- Data Accuracy: AI can enhance data accuracy by identifying and correcting errors in patient records, improving the reliability of health information systems.

By leveraging these AI capabilities, healthcare systems can significantly improve the quality of care, ensuring that it is safe, effective, patient-centered, timely, efficient, and equitable.

6.5 Addressing the issue of Healthcare Workforce Shortages

AI can play a significant role in addressing healthcare workforce shortages by enhancing efficiency, supporting education and training, optimizing resource allocation, and reducing the burden on healthcare professionals. Here are some ways AI can help mitigate the key drivers and impacts of healthcare workforce shortages:

Key Drivers of Healthcare Workforce Shortages

1. Aging Population and Workforce

- Predictive Analytics: AI can forecast healthcare demand based on population aging trends, helping to plan and allocate resources effectively.
- Robotic Assistance: AI-driven robots can assist with routine tasks, allowing healthcare professionals to focus on more complex care needs and extending the capacity of the current workforce.

2. Increasing Healthcare Demand

- Automated Diagnostics: AI can streamline diagnostics by analysing medical images, lab results, and patient data, reducing the time needed for healthcare professionals to diagnose and treat conditions.
- Chronic Disease Management: AI can support the management of chronic diseases through remote monitoring and personalized treatment plans, reducing the workload on healthcare providers.

3. Training and Education Gaps

- Virtual Training: AI-powered virtual reality (VR) and augmented reality (AR) platforms can provide immersive training experiences, improving the quality and efficiency of healthcare education.
- Adaptive Learning: AI can create personalized learning paths for healthcare students, addressing individual gaps in knowledge and ensuring a more competent workforce.

4. Geographic and Specialty Maldistribution

- Telehealth Services: AI-driven telehealth platforms can extend the reach of healthcare services to rural and underserved areas, providing access to specialists and primary care providers remotely.

- Resource Allocation: AI can optimize the distribution of healthcare professionals across regions and specialties by analysing demand and supply data, ensuring a more balanced workforce distribution.

5. Burnout and Job Satisfaction

- Administrative Automation: AI can automate administrative tasks such as scheduling, billing, and record-keeping, reducing the administrative burden on healthcare professionals.
- Mental Health Support: AI-driven mental health apps and virtual assistants can provide support to healthcare workers, helping to manage stress and prevent burnout.

Impacts of Healthcare Workforce Shortages

1. Reduced Access to Care

- Virtual Care: AI can facilitate virtual consultations and remote monitoring, increasing access to care for patients in areas with workforce shortages.
- Efficient Triage: AI can prioritize patient cases based on urgency, ensuring that those in most need receive timely care.

2. Lower Quality of Care

- Clinical Decision Support: AI can provide real-time decision support to healthcare professionals, enhancing the quality of care by offering evidence-based recommendations and reducing the likelihood of errors.
- Performance Monitoring: AI can continuously monitor healthcare delivery and provide feedback to healthcare professionals, helping to maintain high standards of care.

3. Increased Healthcare Costs

- Operational Efficiency: AI can optimize hospital operations, including staffing, supply chain management, and patient flow, reducing costs associated with workforce shortages.

- Cost-Effective Solutions: AI can identify cost-effective treatment options and resource allocation strategies, helping to manage healthcare expenditures.

4. Public Health Risks

- Surveillance and Response: AI can enhance public health surveillance by analysing data from various sources to detect potential outbreaks early and coordinate response efforts.
- Emergency Management: AI can assist in planning and managing public health emergencies, ensuring that resources are used efficiently and effectively during crises.

By leveraging AI, healthcare systems can address the multifaceted issue of workforce shortages, ultimately improving the quality, accessibility, and sustainability of care.

6.6 Addressing the issue of avoidable healthcare cost

AI can contribute significantly to mitigating the issue of healthcare cost increases in several ways:

Efficiency Improvements: AI can optimize various healthcare processes, including administrative tasks, resource allocation, and supply chain management. By automating repetitive tasks, reducing errors, and streamlining workflows, AI helps healthcare organizations operate more efficiently, thereby reducing costs associated with inefficiencies driven by profit motives or market competition.

Preventive Care and Early Intervention: AI algorithms can analyse large datasets to identify individuals at high risk of developing chronic conditions or experiencing adverse health events. By proactively targeting preventive interventions and early treatment, healthcare providers can reduce the overall burden of disease and associated healthcare costs over time.

Remote Monitoring and Telehealth: AI-enabled remote monitoring devices and telehealth platforms allow patients to receive care from the comfort of their homes, reducing the need for costly hospital visits and readmissions. By remotely monitoring patients' health metrics and providing virtual consultations, healthcare providers can intervene early to prevent complications and reduce healthcare expenditures.

Healthcare Fraud Detection: AI algorithms can analyse large volumes of healthcare claims data to identify patterns indicative of fraudulent activities, such as billing for unnecessary services or upcoding. By detecting and preventing healthcare fraud, AI helps safeguard healthcare funds and ensures that resources are allocated efficiently.

Price Transparency: AI-powered tools can analyse healthcare pricing data to provide patients with greater transparency regarding the cost of medical services, procedures, and treatments. By empowering patients to make informed decisions about their healthcare based on cost considerations, AI promotes competition among healthcare providers to offer more affordable and value-driven services.

Drug Utilization Reviews (DUR): AI-driven DUR platforms can analyse prescribing patterns within healthcare organizations to identify opportunities for optimization, cost containment, and quality improvement. By evaluating medication utilization metrics, adherence rates, and therapeutic outcomes, AI helps healthcare providers align prescribing behaviours with best practices and organizational priorities.

6.7 Addressing the issue of Data Deluge

Artificial intelligence offers a powerful solution to address the challenges posed by the exponential expansion of healthcare data. Here's how AI can help:

Data Processing and Analysis: AI techniques, such as machine learning and natural language processing, can automate the process of sifting through large volumes of healthcare data to identify patterns, correlations, and trends. AI algorithms can quickly analyse diverse data sources, including EHRs, medical imaging, genetic data, and wearable device data, to extract valuable insights that would be difficult or time-consuming for humans to uncover.

Predictive Analytics: AI can leverage historical healthcare data to develop predictive models that forecast patient outcomes, disease progression, and healthcare resource utilization. These predictive analytics tools enable healthcare providers to anticipate patient needs, identify at-risk populations, and allocate resources more efficiently to improve patient outcomes and reduce costs.

Personalized Medicine: AI algorithms can analyse individual patient data, such as genetic information, medical history, and lifestyle factors, to tailor treatments and interventions to each patient's unique characteristics and needs. By enabling personalized medicine approaches, AI can improve treatment efficacy, minimize adverse effects, and enhance patient satisfaction.

Decision Support Systems: AI-powered decision support systems can assist healthcare providers in making more informed clinical decisions by synthesizing relevant patient data, medical literature, and best practices. These systems can provide real-time recommendations for diagnosis, treatment planning, and medication selection, ultimately improving patient care quality and safety.

Data Integration and Interoperability: AI technologies can facilitate the integration of heterogeneous healthcare data from disparate sources by standardizing formats, reconciling terminology differences, and enabling interoperability between systems. AI-driven data integration solutions streamline the process of aggregating and harmonizing data for analysis, enhancing the efficiency and accuracy of healthcare data management.

Privacy and Security: AI algorithms can help safeguard patient privacy and data security by implementing robust encryption, access control, and anonymization techniques. AI-driven privacy-preserving methods enable healthcare organizations to comply with regulatory requirements such as HIPAA, GDPR, DISHA and other data protection laws while still leveraging the full potential of healthcare data for analysis and innovation.

Research Acceleration: AI accelerates medical research by automating tasks such as literature review, data mining, and hypothesis generation. AI-powered research tools enable scientists to explore vast datasets, discover novel insights, and expedite the translation of research findings into clinical practice, driving medical innovation and improving patient outcomes.

6.8 Addressing Administrative Burden in Healthcare

AI can significantly alleviate administrative burdens in healthcare by streamlining documentation, ensuring regulatory compliance, optimizing prior authorizations, enhancing billing and coding processes, and improving patient coordination. Here's how AI addresses these specific areas:

Types of Administrative Burden in Healthcare

1. Documentation Requirements

- Automated Data Entry: AI-powered tools can automate the entry of patient information into electronic health records (EHRs), reducing the time healthcare providers spend on documentation.
- Natural Language Processing (NLP): AI with NLP capabilities can transcribe and interpret clinical notes, converting spoken or handwritten notes into structured data in real-time.
- Template and Voice Recognition: AI can use templates and voice recognition software to pre-fill forms and documentation, making it quicker for providers to complete required paperwork.

2. Regulatory Compliance

- Compliance Monitoring: AI can continuously monitor healthcare practices to ensure compliance with regulations and Medicare requirements, alerting staff to potential issues before they become violations.

- Automated Reporting: AI can generate reports required for regulatory compliance automatically, reducing the manual effort involved in preparing and submitting these documents.

3. Prior Authorizations

- Streamlined Workflows: AI can automate the process of obtaining prior authorizations by extracting necessary patient information from EHRs and submitting it to insurance companies for approval.
- Predictive Approvals: AI can predict the likelihood of approval for certain treatments based on historical data, helping providers make informed decisions and reducing the need for re-submissions.

4. Billing and Coding

- Automated Coding: AI can analyse clinical notes and automatically assign appropriate ICD-10 and CPT codes, ensuring accuracy and reducing the time spent on manual coding.
- Error Detection: AI can identify and correct errors in billing codes before claims are submitted, reducing the likelihood of denials and the need for resubmission.

5. Patient Coordination

- Care Coordination Platforms: AI can facilitate seamless communication and data sharing between different healthcare providers, ensuring that patient information is up-to-date and accessible.
- Automated Referrals: AI can manage referrals by automatically identifying and contacting appropriate specialists, scheduling appointments, and sharing relevant medical records.

Causes of Administrative Burden in Healthcare

1. Complexity of Regulations

- Regulation Simplification: AI can help interpret and simplify complex regulations, providing healthcare providers with clear guidelines and reducing confusion.
- Automated Updates: AI systems can keep track of regulatory changes and update compliance protocols automatically, ensuring that healthcare providers are always in line with current regulations.

2. Fragmented Systems

- Interoperability Solutions: AI can bridge gaps between different EHR systems, facilitating data exchange and reducing the need for duplicate data entry.
- Unified Dashboards: AI can create unified dashboards that integrate data from various sources, providing a comprehensive view of patient information and reducing administrative redundancy.

3. Insurance Requirements

- Standardized Documentation: AI can standardize documentation processes across different insurance plans, reducing variability and simplifying compliance with insurance requirements.
- Real-Time Verification: AI can perform real-time insurance verification, ensuring that all necessary documentation is complete and accurate before submission.

4. Resource Constraints

- Resource Optimization: AI can optimize the allocation of administrative tasks, ensuring that staff time is used efficiently and effectively.
- AI Assistants: AI-driven virtual assistants can support smaller practices by handling routine administrative tasks, allowing healthcare professionals to focus on patient care.

Impacts of Administrative Burden in Healthcare

1. Provider Burnout

- Workload Reduction: By automating repetitive tasks, AI reduces the administrative workload on healthcare providers, helping to alleviate burnout and increase job satisfaction.
- Task Prioritization: AI can prioritize administrative tasks, ensuring that critical items are addressed first and allowing providers to spend more time with patients.

2. Patient Care

- Improved Efficiency: AI streamlines administrative processes, enabling healthcare providers to dedicate more time to direct patient care, which can lead to better health outcomes.
- Faster Decision-Making: AI can provide real-time access to patient information and insights, supporting quicker and more informed clinical decisions.

3. Healthcare Costs

- Cost Reduction: Automating administrative tasks reduces the need for additional administrative staff and decreases the time spent on non-clinical activities, lowering overall healthcare costs.
- Efficiency Gains: AI improves operational efficiency, reducing waste and saving resources that can be redirected to patient care.

4. Access to Care

- Reduced Delays: By streamlining processes like prior authorizations and insurance verifications, AI reduces delays in patient care, ensuring timely access to necessary treatments.
- Enhanced Coordination: AI improves care coordination, facilitating smoother transitions between different providers and reducing the administrative barriers that can delay care.

By leveraging AI, healthcare systems can significantly reduce administrative burdens, leading to more efficient operations, better patient care, and improved job satisfaction for healthcare providers.

6.9 Addressing the Pharmaceutical Issues

AI can address the **Pharmaceutical Issues**issues related to drug pricing and the availability of medications through various innovative approaches, enhancing transparency, optimizing production, and improving supply chain management. Here's a detailed explanation of how AI can tackle these challenges:

Addressing Drug Pricing

1. Research and Development (R&D) Costs

- AI-Driven Drug Discovery: AI can analyse vast datasets to identify potential drug candidates faster and more accurately than traditional methods. This reduces the time and cost associated with R&D by predicting which compounds are likely to succeed in clinical trials.
- Virtual Screening and Simulation: AI can simulate drug interactions at the molecular level, predicting efficacy and toxicity, thus streamlining the preclinical phase and reducing the number of compounds that need to be physically tested.

2. Patent Protections

- Patent Analytics: AI can analyse patent databases to identify opportunities for developing generic versions of drugs whose patents are expiring, promoting competition and reducing prices.
- Innovation Incentives: AI can help design new drug formulations or delivery methods that bypass existing patents, fostering innovation while providing more affordable options.

3. Marketing and Sales Expenses

- Targeted Marketing Strategies: AI can optimize marketing strategies by analysing healthcare provider prescribing patterns and patient demographics, reducing the need for extensive marketing budgets.
- Sales Forecasting: AI can predict market demand more accurately, helping pharmaceutical companies allocate resources more efficiently and reduce unnecessary spending.

4. Lack of Price Regulation

- Price Transparency Tools: AI can create platforms that compare drug prices across different pharmacies and regions, empowering consumers and healthcare providers to make cost-effective decisions.
- Regulatory Compliance: AI can help regulators monitor drug prices and ensure compliance with pricing regulations, identifying unjustified price hikes and monopolistic practices.

Impact on Patient Access

1. Financial Barriers

- Personalized Financial Assistance: AI can identify patients who need financial assistance and connect them with relevant programs, reducing the financial burden of high drug costs.
- Insurance Optimization: AI can assist patients in selecting insurance plans that provide the best coverage for their medication needs, ensuring they have access to necessary treatments.

2. Influence on Prescribing Behaviours

- Clinical Decision Support: AI-driven tools can provide evidence-based recommendations to healthcare providers, highlighting cost-effective alternatives and reducing the influence of pharmaceutical marketing on prescribing decisions.

- Formulary Optimization: AI can help insurers and healthcare providers design formularies that prioritize cost-effective and clinically effective medications.

3. Health Disparities

- Access to Information: AI can disseminate information about low-cost drug alternatives, discount programs, and generic options, reducing health disparities and improving access to essential medications.
- Targeted Interventions: AI can identify underserved populations and regions with limited access to affordable medications, enabling targeted interventions to address these gaps.

Addressing Availability of Medications

Drug Shortages

1. Manufacturing Issues

- Predictive Maintenance: AI can monitor manufacturing equipment and processes in real-time, predicting failures and maintenance needs to prevent production delays.
- Quality Control: AI can enhance quality control by analysing production data and detecting anomalies early, reducing the risk of manufacturing issues that lead to drug shortages.

2. Regulatory Challenges

- Streamlined Approval Processes: AI can assist regulatory bodies by analysing data more efficiently, accelerating the approval of manufacturing changes and new suppliers.
- Compliance Monitoring: AI can ensure continuous compliance with regulatory standards, minimizing delays due to regulatory issues.

3. Market Dynamics

- Economic Analysis: AI can analyse market trends and predict which drugs are at risk of being discontinued, enabling proactive measures to ensure their continued availability.
- Alternative Production Strategies: AI can identify opportunities for producing low-profit-margin drugs more cost-effectively, ensuring their availability despite economic challenges.

4. Global Supply Chain Dependencies

- Supply Chain Optimization: AI can optimize supply chain logistics by predicting demand, identifying bottlenecks, and coordinating supply chain activities to ensure timely delivery of raw materials and finished products.
- Risk Management: AI can assess geopolitical risks, natural disasters, and other factors affecting global supply chains, enabling proactive measures to mitigate these risks.

Impact on Patient Care

1. Treatment Delays

- Real-Time Inventory Management: AI can monitor drug inventories in real-time, predicting shortages and enabling timely restocking to prevent treatment delays.
- Dynamic Resource Allocation: AI can optimize the allocation of resources during shortages, ensuring that critical medications are available where they are needed most.

2. Use of Alternatives

- Alternative Treatment Analysis: AI can analyse the efficacy and safety profiles of alternative medications, providing healthcare providers with evidence-based recommendations to ensure optimal patient care.
- Supply Chain Resilience: AI can enhance the resilience of supply chains, ensuring that alternative medications are readily available in case of shortages.

3. Increased Costs

- Cost Prediction and Management: AI can predict cost increases due to drug shortages and help healthcare systems manage these costs more effectively.
- Efficient Procurement: AI can optimize procurement strategies, securing better prices for alternative medications and reducing the financial impact on patients and healthcare systems.

By leveraging AI, the pharmaceutical industry can address the high costs and availability issues of medications, ensuring that patients have access to affordable and necessary treatments, thereby improving overall healthcare outcomes.

Chapter 07

AI IN HEALTHCARE OPERATIONS

Healthcare operations management is the discipline focused on supervising and enhancing the nonclinical functions within a healthcare organization. It encompasses a range of activities, including managing the physical facilities, deployment and supervising staff, allocating and controlling the budget, interacting with external stake holders like insurance companies and suppliers, integrating technology, ensuring regulatory compliance, and facilitating effective internal communication and coordination. The goal is to enhance the efficiency, effectiveness, and quality of healthcare services.

One of the primary benefits of automation is the enhancement of operational efficiency. Automated systems can handle repetitive tasks, such as scheduling appointments, processing insurance claims, and managing inventory, with greater speed and accuracy than manual processes. This efficiency not only reduces the administrative burden on healthcare staff but also allows them to focus more on direct patient care. As a result, patients experience shorter wait times and more timely access to services.

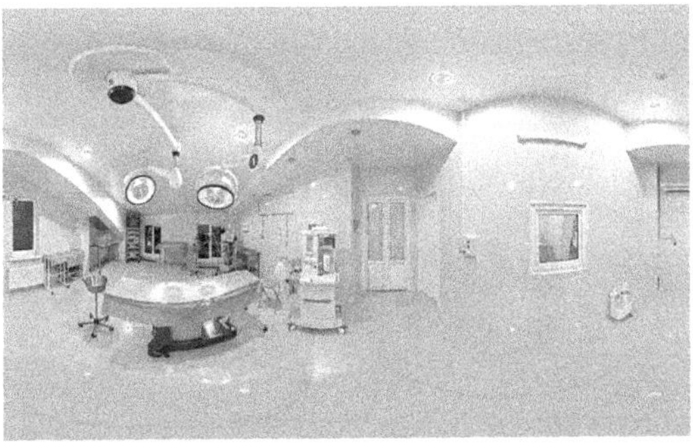

Human errors in administrative functions like data entry can lead to a range of serious issues, including incorrect billing, treatment delays, and potential legal complications. Automation has emerged as a powerful solution to address these challenges. By implementing automated systems, healthcare facilities can significantly reduce errors, enhance the quality of care, and lower operational costs.

Automation enhances the precision of administrative tasks, which boosts overall productivity. For example, automated billing systems help ensure accurate invoicing, minimizing the need for time-consuming dispute resolution. Similarly, automated scheduling tools can reduce the rate of missed appointments, optimizing the efficiency of healthcare staff and improving patient care. This shift allows human resources to concentrate on direct patient interactions and other critical tasks, further elevating the standard of care.

Artificial intelligence has the potential to significantly enhance healthcare operations by streamlining and improving various tasks. With the global healthcare AI market surpassing $15.4 billion USD in 2022 and projected to grow rapidly with an expectation of reaching $148 billion USD by 2029, its impact on healthcare operations management is becoming increasingly evident. AI's ability to optimize administrative workflows and boost back-office efficiency represents one of its most immediate and valuable contributions to the field. As AI technologies advance, they are poised to transform how healthcare facilities manage their operations, leading to more efficient and effective administrative processes.

Following are some impact of AI integration in Healthcare administration

1. Utilize staff and equipment efficiently
2. Dispatch mobile workers efficiently
3. Streamline internal communication
4. Improve patient communication
5. Reduce manual administrative work
6. Manage health insurance claims
7. Recruit excellent employees

7.1 Schedule staff and equipment efficiently

In the evolving landscape of healthcare, the integration of artificial intelligence offers transformative benefits, particularly in the efficient utilization of staff and equipment. AI technologies are increasingly being leveraged to optimize resource management, leading to significant improvements in operational efficiency and patient care.

1. Optimizing Staff Allocation

AI-powered tools can analyse vast amounts of data to forecast patient needs, manage staff schedules, and ensure optimal coverage. For instance, predictive analytics can anticipate peak times in patient flow, allowing healthcare facilities to adjust staffing levels proactively. By analysing patterns and trends, AI can help allocate staff where they are most needed, reducing overstaffing during quieter periods and preventing understaffing during high-demand times. This not only enhances the quality of care by ensuring adequate staffing levels but also improves staff satisfaction by reducing burnout and stress.

2. Enhancing Equipment Utilization

Efficient equipment management is crucial in healthcare settings, where costly and specialized devices are often underutilized. AI can help track and manage equipment usage by monitoring real-time data on device performance and availability. For example, AI systems can schedule and coordinate the use of diagnostic machines, surgical instruments, and other critical equipment, ensuring that these resources are used to their fullest potential without unnecessary delays. This leads to better equipment turnover rates, reduced downtime, and overall improved operational efficiency.

3. Streamlining Workflow Processes

AI-driven systems can automate routine tasks such as scheduling, inventory management, and equipment maintenance. Automated scheduling tools can match the availability of providers and equipment, ensuring that appointments are optimized and resources are allocated effectively. Similarly, AI can manage inventory by predicting supply needs based on historical data and current usage trends, preventing shortages or overstock situations.

4. Improving Coordination between Staff and Equipment

Effective communication and coordination between healthcare staff and the use of equipment are critical for delivering high-quality care. AI systems can facilitate this by providing real-time updates and alerts about equipment status and availability. For example, if a piece of equipment is in use or undergoing maintenance, AI can notify the relevant staff members, ensuring that they can plan and adjust their activities accordingly.

5. Reducing Operational Costs

By optimizing the use of both staff and equipment, AI can lead to substantial cost savings. Efficient resource management reduces waste and minimizes the need for additional equipment or staff. Additionally, improved scheduling and inventory management help avoid unnecessary expenses related to idle equipment or overstaffed shifts.

6. Enhancing Patient Outcomes

When staff and equipment are utilized efficiently, the overall quality of patient care improves. Reduced wait times, better resource availability, and timely interventions contribute to more positive patient experiences and outcomes. AI's role in optimizing these factors ensures that patients receive timely and appropriate care, which can lead to faster recovery and higher satisfaction.

7.2 Dispatch mobile workers efficiently

The integration of artificial intelligence in healthcare is revolutionizing the way mobile workers—such as home health nurses, paramedics, and medical technicians—are managed and deployed. Efficient dispatch of these professionals is crucial for optimizing patient care, improving operational efficiency, and reducing costs. AI technologies are enhancing this aspect of healthcare operations in several transformative ways.

1. Real-Time Resource Allocation

AI systems can analyse real-time data to determine the optimal deployment of mobile workers based on current needs and locations. By processing information such as patient urgency, worker availability, and geographic location, AI can make dynamic decisions on where to send mobile staff. This ensures that healthcare professionals are dispatched to the most critical cases first, improving response times and patient outcomes.

2. Predictive Analytics for Demand Forecasting

AI utilizes predictive analytics to anticipate future demand for mobile healthcare services. By analysing historical data, trends, and external factors such as seasonal illness outbreaks or demographic changes, AI can forecast periods of high demand. This allows healthcare organizations to proactively schedule and deploy mobile workers, ensuring that there are enough professionals available during peak times and avoiding shortages during critical periods.

3. Route Optimization

AI-powered route optimization tools can significantly enhance the efficiency of mobile worker dispatch. By calculating the fastest and most efficient routes to patient locations, AI can reduce travel time and fuel consumption. This not only speeds up response times but also helps in managing costs and reducing the environmental impact of healthcare operations. Real-time traffic data integration further enhances route planning by avoiding delays caused by road conditions or traffic jams.

4. Dynamic Scheduling and Adjustments

AI systems can adapt schedules in real-time based on emerging needs and changing circumstances. For example, if an urgent case arises or if a scheduled appointment is canceled, AI can quickly reassign mobile workers to ensure that resources are used effectively. This flexibility helps maintain a balance between scheduled tasks and unexpected demands, ensuring that patient needs are consistently met.

5. Enhanced Communication and Coordination

AI facilitates improved communication between mobile workers and central management. Mobile workers can receive real-time updates, alerts, and instructions through AI-driven platforms. These systems can also provide critical information such as patient history, required interventions, and necessary equipment, enabling mobile staff to be fully prepared before arriving at a patient's location. Enhanced communication ensures that mobile workers can perform their duties more effectively and with greater accuracy.

6. Data-Driven Performance Monitoring

AI tools can monitor and analyse the performance of mobile workers, providing insights into productivity, efficiency, and areas for improvement. By evaluating metrics such as response times, patient feedback, and task completion rates, AI can help healthcare organizations identify best practices and address any inefficiencies. This data-driven approach supports continuous improvement in service delivery and resource management.

7. Cost Efficiency

Efficient dispatching of mobile workers through AI leads to cost savings by reducing unnecessary travel, optimizing resource allocation, and improving overall operational efficiency. By minimizing idle time and ensuring that mobile staff are deployed effectively, healthcare organizations can achieve better financial management and allocate resources where they are most needed.

7.3 Streamline healthcare operations communications

Effective communication within healthcare operations is crucial for ensuring seamless coordination among healthcare professionals, enhancing patient care, and maintaining operational efficiency. The integration of artificial intelligence into healthcare communications offers transformative benefits, enabling more streamlined, efficient, and accurate exchanges of information across various levels of the healthcare system.

1. Centralized Communication Platforms

AI facilitates the creation of centralized communication platforms that integrate various forms of communication, including messaging, email, and alerts, into a single interface. These platforms enable healthcare staff to access and manage all communication channels from one place, reducing the risk of missed messages or fragmented information. Centralized systems streamline communication, making it easier for healthcare professionals to collaborate and share critical information.

2. Automated Information Routing:

AI-driven systems can automatically route communications to the appropriate recipients based on predefined criteria. For instance, if a patient's test results are ready, the AI system can ensure that the results are sent directly to the relevant healthcare provider, patient, or specialist. This reduces the likelihood of delays and ensures that the right people receive the right information at the right time.

3. Enhanced Coordination and Collaboration:

AI tools can improve coordination among healthcare teams by facilitating real-time updates and notifications. For example, if there is a change in a patient's status or a new development in a care plan, AI can instantly notify all relevant team members. This ensures that everyone involved in the patient's care is up-to-date with the latest information, leading to more effective collaboration and decision-making.

4. Natural Language Processing (NLP) for Improved Communication:

Natural Language Processing (NLP), a subset of AI, can analyse and interpret human language to improve communication. NLP can be used to transcribe and summarize conversations, extract key information from unstructured data, and even generate reports or documentation automatically. This reduces the burden of manual data entry and documentation, allowing healthcare professionals to focus more on patient care.

5. Predictive Analytics for Communication Needs:

AI systems can use predictive analytics to anticipate communication needs based on historical data and current trends. For example, if a particular type of communication is frequently required during certain times of the day or in specific scenarios, AI can preemptively prepare and send relevant information or alerts. This proactive approach helps in managing communication more effectively and reducing the risk of missed or delayed information.

6. Improved Patient Engagement:

AI enhances patient communication by providing automated and personalized interactions. Chatbots and virtual assistants can handle routine inquiries, schedule appointments, and provide patients with information about their care plans. This not only improves patient engagement by providing timely responses but also frees up healthcare staff to focus on more complex tasks and direct patient interactions.

7. Secure and Compliant Communication:

AI can ensure that all communications adhere to regulatory requirements and privacy standards. Automated systems can manage and monitor data security protocols, encrypt sensitive information, and ensure that communications comply with various governmental and other regulations across the world. This enhances the security and confidentiality of patient information, reducing the risk of data breaches.

8. Real-Time Translation Services:

AI-powered translation tools can break down language barriers by providing real-time translation services for non-English speaking patients and staff. This ensures that language differences do not hinder effective communication and helps in delivering equitable care to diverse patient populations.

9. Performance Monitoring and Optimization:

AI can track and analyse communication patterns and performance metrics, providing insights into areas where communication processes can be improved. By identifying bottlenecks or inefficiencies, AI helps healthcare organizations optimize their communication strategies, leading to more efficient operations and better overall performance.

7.4 Improve patient communication

Effective patient communication is a cornerstone of high-quality healthcare, impacting everything from patient satisfaction to treatment outcomes. The integration of artificial intelligence into healthcare communication practices has the potential to significantly enhance interactions between patients and healthcare providers, making these interactions more efficient, personalized, and supportive.

1. Personalized Patient Interactions

AI enables the creation of personalized communication experiences by analyzing patient data, including medical history, preferences, and past interactions. AI-driven systems can tailor messages and recommendations to individual patients, making communication more relevant and engaging. For example, automated systems can send personalized appointment reminders, health tips, and follow-up instructions based on a patient's specific health conditions and treatment plans.

2. Automated Appointment Scheduling and Reminders:

AI-powered scheduling tools simplify the appointment booking process for patients by providing user-friendly interfaces for selecting available times, rescheduling, or canceling appointments. Additionally, automated reminder systems use AI to send timely notifications via email, SMS, or app alerts, reducing the likelihood of missed appointments and helping patients adhere to their care plans. This reduces administrative burden and improves patient compliance.

3. Virtual Health Assistants:

AI-driven virtual assistants or chatbots are available 24/7 to assist patients with a range of tasks, from answering common questions about symptoms and treatment options to providing information about healthcare services. These virtual assistants can offer immediate responses and support, enhancing patient experience and reducing the need for direct interaction with human staff for routine queries. This ensures that patients have access to timely information whenever they need it.

4. Enhanced Remote Monitoring and Support:

AI technologies facilitate remote patient monitoring by collecting and analysing data from wearable devices and health apps. This data can be used to provide real-time feedback to patients about their health status, track adherence to treatment plans, and identify potential issues before they become serious. Patients receive continuous support and guidance, which helps in managing chronic conditions and improving overall health outcomes.

5. Improved Health Literacy:

AI tools can aid in improving patient health literacy by delivering clear, accessible information about medical conditions, treatment options, and self-care practices. AI-driven educational platforms can break down complex medical terminology into understandable language and provide visual aids or interactive content to enhance comprehension. This empowers patients to make informed decisions about their health and treatment.

6. Multilingual Communication:

AI-powered translation and language processing tools address language barriers by providing real-time translation services. These tools help in delivering accurate and culturally sensitive communication to non-English speaking patients, ensuring that language differences do not impede access to healthcare information and services. This fosters better understanding and engagement across diverse patient populations.

7. Proactive Health Management:

AI systems can use predictive analytics to anticipate patient needs and provide proactive communication. For instance, AI can analyze data to identify patients at risk of developing certain conditions and proactively reach out with preventive care recommendations or early intervention strategies. This proactive approach helps in managing health more effectively and preventing complications.

8. Real-Time Feedback and Support:

AI can facilitate real-time feedback mechanisms where patients can share their experiences, concerns, or symptoms instantly. This immediate feedback allows healthcare providers to address issues quickly and make necessary adjustments to care plans. AI can also analyse patient feedback to identify common concerns and areas for improvement, enhancing overall patient satisfaction.

9. Data-Driven Insights for Personalized Care:

AI analyses patient interactions and outcomes to provide healthcare providers with valuable insights into patient preferences and communication effectiveness. This data helps in refining communication strategies, tailoring patient interactions, and improving overall engagement. By understanding patient behaviours and responses, healthcare providers can better align their communication practices with patient needs.

10. Efficient Management of Patient Inquiries:

AI-driven systems can handle and prioritize patient inquiries efficiently, directing them to the appropriate departments or professionals based on the nature of the request. This ensures that patients receive timely and accurate responses, reducing wait times and improving the efficiency of the healthcare system.

7.5 Reduce manual administrative work

Manual administrative tasks in healthcare, such as data entry, scheduling, and billing, are time-consuming and prone to errors, which can detract from patient care and operational efficiency. The integration of artificial intelligence in healthcare administration offers a transformative approach to reducing these manual tasks, leading to increased accuracy, efficiency, and overall effectiveness in healthcare operations.

1. Automating Routine Data Entry

One of the most significant impacts of AI in healthcare administration is the automation of routine data entry tasks. AI systems equipped with Optical Character Recognition (OCR) and Natural Language Processing (NLP) can extract and input data from various sources, such as handwritten notes, digital forms, and electronic health records (EHRs). This automation reduces the need for manual data entry, minimizes errors, and frees up administrative staff to focus on more complex and patient-centric tasks.

2. Streamlining Appointment Scheduling

AI-driven scheduling tools can automate the process of managing appointments, coordinating availability, and rescheduling. These systems use algorithms to match patient needs with provider availability, handle appointment confirmations, and send reminders to patients. By reducing the manual effort involved in scheduling, AI enhances efficiency, reduces the risk of double-bookings, and improves the overall patient experience.

3. Simplifying Billing and Coding

Billing and coding are complex processes that require accuracy and attention to detail. AI can automate the coding of diagnoses and procedures based on clinical documentation, reducing the risk of errors and ensuring compliance with billing regulations. AI systems can also handle claims submission, track reimbursements, and manage denials, significantly reducing the administrative burden on billing staff and accelerating the revenue cycle.

4. Enhancing Workflow Management

AI can optimize various administrative workflows by automating routine tasks such as processing referrals, managing patient intake, and handling insurance verification. For example, AI systems can automatically verify insurance coverage and eligibility, reducing the need for manual verification and minimizing delays in patient care. By streamlining these workflows, AI improves operational efficiency and accelerates administrative processes.

5. Improving Document Management

AI technologies can assist in managing and organizing vast amounts of documentation within healthcare facilities. Intelligent document management systems can categorize, index, and retrieve documents based on content, making it easier for administrative staff to access and manage records. AI-driven tools can also facilitate document sharing and collabouration, enhancing efficiency and reducing the time spent on manual document handling.

6. Automating Reporting and Analytics

AI can generate and analyse reports automatically, providing valuable insights into operational performance, patient outcomes, and financial metrics. By automating the generation of reports and analysing data trends, AI reduces the manual effort required to compile and interpret information. This allows healthcare organizations to make data-driven decisions more quickly and accurately.

7. Enhancing Patient Registration

AI-driven systems can automate the patient registration process by collecting and verifying patient information through online forms and digital interfaces. These systems can also handle eligibility checks and integrate with EHRs to update patient records automatically. By reducing the manual effort involved in registration, AI streamlines the patient onboarding process and improves data accuracy.

8. Reducing Error Rates

Manual administrative tasks are susceptible to human errors, which can lead to complications such as incorrect billing, delayed appointments, and inaccurate patient records. AI systems, with their ability to process data accurately and consistently, reduce the likelihood of errors. This leads to improved data integrity, fewer administrative mistakes, and a more reliable healthcare operation.

9. Improving Compliance and Regulation

AI can help ensure compliance with healthcare regulations and standards by automating tasks related to documentation and reporting. AI systems can monitor adherence to regulatory requirements, generate compliance reports, and alert staff to potential issues. This reduces the administrative burden associated with compliance and helps maintain high standards of care.

10. Supporting Staff Efficiency

By automating routine administrative tasks, AI allows healthcare staff to focus on more value-added activities, such as direct patient care and complex problem-solving. This shift not only enhances staff productivity but also improves job satisfaction by reducing the monotonous and repetitive aspects of administrative work.

7.6 Manage health insurance claims

The management of health insurance claims is a critical component of healthcare administration that directly affects the financial stability of healthcare organizations and the satisfaction of patients. Traditional processes for handling insurance claims can be cumbersome, prone to errors, and time-consuming. The integration of artificial intelligence into this aspect of healthcare offers transformative improvements, enhancing accuracy, efficiency, and overall effectiveness in claims management.

1. Automating Claims Processing:

AI-driven systems can automate the entire claims processing workflow, from submission to reimbursement. These systems use algorithms to review and validate claims based on predefined rules and criteria. Automated processing reduces the manual effort required for tasks such as data entry, claims adjudication, and follow-up, leading to faster turnaround times and fewer delays in payment.

2. Improving Accuracy with Data Validation:

AI enhances the accuracy of claims management by performing real-time data validation. AI systems can cross-check submitted claims against patient records, insurance policies, and billing codes to identify discrepancies or errors. By flagging potential issues before claims are submitted or processed, AI helps reduce the likelihood of rejections, denials, and the need for resubmissions.

3. Streamlining Claims Adjudication:

Claims adjudication involves evaluating and deciding the validity of insurance claims based on policy coverage and medical necessity. AI can streamline this process by analysing claims data and applying complex algorithms to determine the appropriate reimbursement amounts. This speeds up adjudication, reduces administrative overhead, and ensures that claims are handled consistently and fairly.

4. Detecting Fraud and Abuse:

AI systems can significantly improve the detection of fraudulent claims and billing abuse. By analysing patterns in claims data, AI can identify anomalies and unusual patterns that may indicate fraudulent activity. Machine learning models can continuously learn from new data and adapt to emerging fraud schemes, enhancing the ability to detect and prevent fraudulent claims more effectively.

5. Enhancing Claims Status Tracking

AI-powered tools provide real-time tracking and updates on the status of insurance claims. Patients and healthcare providers can access information on claim progress, payment statuses, and any issues that may arise. This transparency reduces uncertainty and improves communication between all parties involved, leading to a better overall experience for both providers and patients.

6. Automating Denial Management

When claims are denied, AI systems can automate the management of denial reasons and assist in the appeal process. AI can analyse the reasons for denials, suggest corrective actions, and generate appeal documentation. This reduces the administrative burden associated with managing denials and appeals, improves the likelihood of successful appeals, and accelerates the resolution process.

7. Enhancing Claims Analytics and Reporting

AI provides advanced analytics and reporting capabilities for insurance claims data. By analysing trends, identifying patterns, and generating detailed reports, AI helps healthcare organizations gain insights into claims performance, reimbursement rates, and common issues. These insights support data-driven decision-making and help in optimizing claims management strategies.

8. Facilitating Efficient Documentation and Compliance

AI tools can assist in managing and organizing the documentation required for insurance claims. Automated systems can ensure that all necessary documents are collected, organized, and submitted in accordance with insurance requirements. This improves compliance with regulatory standards and reduces the risk of claim rejections due to incomplete or inaccurate documentation.

9. Improving Patient Experience

AI enhances the patient experience by simplifying the insurance claims process. Automated systems can provide patients with clear, timely information about their claims, including explanations of coverage and payment details. By reducing the complexity and delays associated with claims, AI contributes to higher patient satisfaction and a more positive healthcare experience.

10. Reducing Administrative Costs

By automating and streamlining claims management processes, AI reduces the administrative costs associated with handling insurance claims. The reduction in manual labour, fewer errors, and faster processing times contribute to lower operational expenses and more efficient use of resources within healthcare organizations.

7.7 Identify excellent candidates for open positions

Recruiting and retaining skilled professionals is essential for the success of any healthcare organization. Identifying the right candidates for open positions can be a challenging and resource-intensive process, involving numerous applications and a rigorous vetting process. The integration of artificial intelligence into healthcare recruitment offers significant advantages, transforming the way organizations identify, evaluate, and select top talent. Here's a detailed look at how AI enhances this critical aspect of healthcare operations.

1. Streamlining Resume Screening:

AI-driven tools can automate the initial screening of resumes and applications by using natural language processing (NLP) to analyse and interpret large volumes of candidate data. AI systems can quickly identify key qualifications, skills, and experience relevant to the open position, reducing the time spent manually reviewing resumes. This speeds up the recruitment process and ensures that only the most suitable candidates are shortlisted for further evaluation.

2. Enhancing Candidate Matching:

AI algorithms can match candidates to job openings based on a combination of their skills, experience, and other relevant criteria. By analysing job descriptions and candidate profiles, AI can assess how well candidates align with the requirements of the position. This matching process helps identify candidates who possess the right mix of qualifications and experience, leading to a higher likelihood of finding the best fit for the role.

3. Reducing Bias in Recruitment:

AI systems can be designed to minimize unconscious bias in the recruitment process by focusing solely on objective criteria and qualifications. By evaluating candidates based on their skills, experience, and performance metrics rather than subjective factors, AI helps promote diversity and inclusivity in hiring. This approach ensures that all candidates are evaluated fairly, based on their ability to perform the job effectively.

4. Predicting Candidate Success:

AI can leverage predictive analytics to assess the potential success of candidates in specific roles. By analysing data from previous hires, including their performance metrics and career progression, AI systems can identify patterns and traits that correlate with successful employees. This predictive capability helps in selecting candidates who are more likely to excel in the position and contribute positively to the organization.

5. Automating Interview Scheduling:

AI-powered tools can automate the scheduling of interviews by integrating with calendars and coordinating availability between candidates and interviewers. This automation reduces the administrative burden of managing interview logistics and minimizes scheduling conflicts. Additionally, AI systems can send reminders and updates to both candidates and interviewers, ensuring a smooth and organized interview process.

6. Enhancing Candidate Engagement:

AI-driven chatbots and virtual assistants can enhance candidate engagement throughout the recruitment process. These tools can answer candidate inquiries, provide updates on application status, and offer information about the organization and job roles. By maintaining regular communication and providing timely responses, AI helps keep candidates informed and engaged, improving their overall experience.

7. Analyzing Candidate Data

AI systems can analyse various data points from candidate applications, assessments, and interviews to provide insights into candidate suitability. By evaluating factors such as skills assessments, cultural fit, and behavioural traits, AI can generate detailed reports and recommendations for hiring managers. These insights support informed decision-making and help in selecting candidates who align with both the technical requirements and organizational culture.

8. Improving Job Advertising and Sourcing

AI can optimize job advertising by targeting the right platforms and channels based on where potential candidates are most likely to be found.

AI algorithms can analyse data on candidate behaviour and preferences to recommend the most effective job boards, social media platforms, and professional networks for posting job openings. This targeted approach increases the visibility of job advertisements and attracts high-quality candidates.

9. Enhancing Onboarding and Integration

AI can support the onboarding process by providing new hires with personalized training and orientation materials. AI-driven platforms can assess the training needs of new employees and deliver tailored content that helps them quickly acclimate to their roles. This enhanced onboarding experience helps new hires integrate more smoothly into the organization and start contributing effectively from day one.

10. Continuous Improvement through Data Analytics

AI systems can continuously analyse recruitment data to identify trends, evaluate the effectiveness of hiring strategies, and refine recruitment processes. By tracking metrics such as time-to-fill, candidate quality, and retention rates, AI provides actionable insights for improving recruitment practices and enhancing the overall effectiveness of the hiring process.

Chapter
08

AI INTEGRATION IN HEALTHCARE

In recent years, the integration of artificial intelligence into healthcare has transformed the landscape of medical practice. From streamlining administrative tasks to revolutionizing diagnostics and treatment planning, AI holds immense potential to enhance patient care and outcomes. However, for healthcare professionals, adopting and integrating AI into their practice requires a deliberate approach encompassing strategies, education, and collaboration. Similarly, patients are not merely recipients of care but active participants in their health journeys. Thus, ensuring patient awareness, engagement, and trust in AI-driven healthcare is paramount. This chapter delves into key considerations for healthcare professionals embarking on the journey of incorporating AI into their daily practice as well as explores strategies to empower patients, enhance their understanding of AI, and foster meaningful engagement in medical decisions.

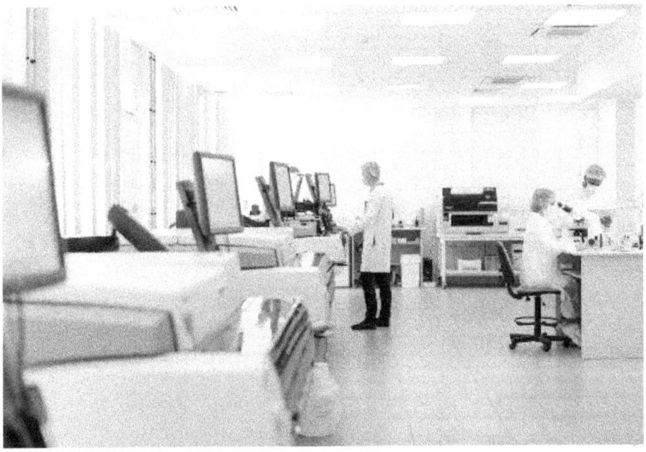

8.1 Strategies to Integrate AI into Healthcare Practice

Adopting AI in healthcare necessitates a strategic approach tailored to the specific needs and constraints of each healthcare setting. Healthcare professionals can employ several strategies to facilitate seamless integration:

1. Needs Assessment: Begin by identifying the areas within healthcare practice where AI can offer the most value. This may involve evaluating existing processes, workflows, and pain points to pinpoint areas ripe for AI intervention

- Analyse Existing Workflows

  Identify Bottlenecks: Look for areas where processes are slow, inefficient, or prone to errors. This could include tasks like image analysis in radiology, administrative tasks like scheduling, or even tasks within drug development.

  Evaluate Workload: Pinpoint areas where healthcare professionals are overloaded or stretched thin. AI can automate repetitive tasks, freeing up valuable time for patient interaction and complex decision-making.

  Consider Patient Needs: Think about areas where patients could benefit from AI-powered tools. This might involve AI-powered chatbots for symptom checkers, medication reminders, or mental health support.

- Leverage Data Analytics

  Data Availability: Identify areas where you have access to rich datasets (electronic health records, imaging scans, etc.). AI thrives on large amounts of data for learning and pattern recognition.

  Data Quality: Ensure the data you have is clean, accurate, and up-to-date. Poor quality data will lead to unreliable AI models.

- Align with Strategic Goals

  Organizational Priorities: Consider how AI can support your healthcare organization's overall goals. This could involve improving patient outcomes, reducing costs, or enhancing operational efficiency.

  Focus on Value: Prioritize AI applications that offer a clear return on investment (ROI) by improving quality, reducing costs, or streamlining processes.

- Benchmarking

  Research Existing Solutions: Look for successful examples of AI implementation in similar healthcare settings. Learn from their experiences and adapt their approaches to your specific needs.

2. Start Small, Scale Up: Implement AI solutions incrementally, starting with pilot projects in low-risk areas. This allows healthcare professionals to assess efficacy, gather feedback, and refine processes before broader implementation. Here's a breakdown of this strategy:

- Identify Low-Risk Areas: Begin by selecting pilot projects or initiatives in low-risk areas of healthcare practice. These could be processes or workflows where the potential impact of AI is significant but the risks associated with implementation are relatively low. For example, implementing AI-driven decision support tools for medication adherence or automating routine administrative tasks like data entry and documentation.
- Proof of Concept: Once a suitable area for AI intervention has been identified, initiate a proof-of-concept or pilot study to test the feasibility and effectiveness of the AI solution. This involves deploying the AI technology in a controlled environment and assessing its performance in real-world scenarios. The proof of concept allows healthcare professionals to validate the AI solution's capabilities, evaluate its impact on clinical workflows, and identify any technical or operational challenges that need to be addressed.

- Gather Feedback and Iterate: Throughout the pilot phase, solicit feedback from healthcare professionals, patients, and other stakeholders involved in the project. Their insights and experiences can provide valuable guidance for refining the AI solution and addressing any usability or functionality issues. By iteratively improving the AI solution based on user feedback, healthcare organizations can enhance its effectiveness and ensure that it meets the needs of end-users.
- Assess Scalability and Sustainability: As the pilot project progresses successfully, assess its scalability and sustainability for broader implementation across the healthcare organization. Consider factors such as resource requirements, infrastructure needs, and organizational readiness to scale up the AI solution effectively. It's essential to develop a roadmap for scaling up the AI initiative while addressing any logistical or operational challenges that may arise.
- Monitor and Measure Impact: Once the AI solution is deployed at scale, monitor its performance and measure its impact on key metrics such as clinical outcomes, workflow efficiency, and patient satisfaction. Continuously evaluate the AI solution's effectiveness in achieving its intended objectives and identify opportunities for further optimization or expansion. By monitoring and measuring the impact of AI integration, healthcare organizations can ensure that it delivers tangible benefits and value to patients and providers alike.

3. Training and Upskilling: Provide comprehensive training programs to healthcare professionals to familiarize them with AI technologies and their applications in clinical practice. This training should cover not only the technical aspects of AI but also its ethical considerations and implications for patient care. Next section of this chapter is allotted exclusively to discuss this point considering the importance of Training and upskilling for the successful integration of AI in healthcare.

4. Embrace Change Management: Recognize that integrating AI may entail organizational changes and cultural shifts. Effective change management strategies, including clear communication, stakeholder engagement, and leadership support, are essential for overcoming resistance and fostering adoption. Here's where effective change management strategies become crucial for ensuring a smooth and successful transition:

- Building a Culture of Open Communication

  Transparency and Early Communication: Clearly communicate the rationale behind AI adoption and its potential benefits for both patients and healthcare professionals. Early and transparent communication reduces anxiety and fosters trust within the organization.

  Open Dialogue: Encourage open dialogue and address any concerns or questions healthcare professionals might have about AI. Actively listen to their feedback and incorporate it into the implementation plan whenever possible.

- Engaging Stakeholders at All Levels

  Leadership Support: Strong leadership support is essential for successful change management. Leaders should champion AI adoption and clearly communicate its importance to achieving organizational goals.

  Multi-disciplinary Teams: Establish multi-disciplinary teams involving healthcare professionals, IT specialists, and administrators. This fosters collaboration and ensures all perspectives are considered throughout the integration process.

- Managing Resistance and Fostering Acceptance

  Understanding Concerns: Acknowledge and address common concerns surrounding AI, such as job displacement or reliance on technology. Focus on how AI can augment human expertise and free up time for more complex tasks.

Success Stories and Recognition: Showcase successful pilot projects and highlight the positive impact of AI on patient care and staff experience. This fosters a sense of ownership and encourages wider acceptance.

- Building Training and Support Structures

  Tailored Training Programs: As discussed earlier, providing comprehensive training programs empowers healthcare professionals with the knowledge and skills to use AI effectively.

  Ongoing Support Systems: Establish ongoing support systems to address questions and concerns that may arise after implementation. This could include dedicated support staff or online resources.

5. Continuous Evaluation and Improvement: Continuously monitor the performance and impact of AI interventions, soliciting feedback from healthcare professionals and patients. This feedback loop enables iterative improvements and ensures that AI solutions remain aligned with evolving healthcare needs.

- Monitoring Performance and Impact: Healthcare organizations should establish mechanisms for monitoring the performance and impact of AI interventions on an ongoing basis. This may involve tracking key performance indicators (KPIs) such as clinical outcomes, workflow efficiency, patient satisfaction, and cost-effectiveness. By systematically collecting and analysing data, organizations can gain insights into the effectiveness of AI solutions and identify areas for improvement.
- Soliciting Feedback: Actively soliciting feedback from healthcare professionals and patients is essential for understanding their experiences with AI technologies. This feedback can

provide valuable insights into the usability, effectiveness, and acceptability of AI solutions in real-world clinical settings. Healthcare organizations can use surveys, focus groups, interviews, and other feedback mechanisms to gather input from stakeholders and incorporate their perspectives into the evaluation process.

- Iterative Improvements: Based on the feedback received, healthcare organizations should prioritize and implement iterative improvements to AI solutions. This may involve addressing usability issues, refining algorithms, optimizing workflows, and enhancing integration with existing systems. By continuously iterating and refining AI technologies based on real-world feedback, organizations can enhance their performance, usability, and impact over time.
- Alignment with Evolving Healthcare Needs: Healthcare needs and priorities are constantly evolving, driven by factors such as advances in medical science, changes in patient demographics, and shifts in regulatory requirements. It's essential for AI solutions to remain aligned with these evolving healthcare needs to ensure their continued relevance and effectiveness. Continuous evaluation and improvement enable organizations to adapt AI technologies to changing circumstances and emerging challenges, ensuring that they continue to deliver value to patients and providers alike.
- Learning from Failures: In addition to successes, organizations should also learn from failures and setbacks encountered during the AI integration process. Failed initiatives can provide valuable lessons about what doesn't work and highlight areas for improvement. By embracing a culture of learning and innovation, organizations can use these experiences to inform future decision-making and avoid repeating past mistakes.

8.2 Training Healthcare Professionals on AI Technologies

Equipping healthcare professionals with the knowledge and skills to harness the potential of AI is paramount for successful integration. Training and education initiatives should encompass the following components:

1. Foundational Understanding: Offer introductory courses that provide healthcare professionals with a foundational understanding of AI concepts, terminology, and principles. Here's what this component should focus on:

Decoding AI Jargon: Many healthcare professionals may not have a background in computer science. This training should break down common AI terms like machine learning, deep learning, algorithms, and neural networks into easily understandable concepts.

AI Fundamentals: The training should introduce core principles of AI, explaining how machines can learn from data and make data-driven predictions. This can involve basic examples of AI applications outside of healthcare to build familiarity.

Interdisciplinary Approach: Given the interdisciplinary nature of AI, it's essential to incorporate insights from computer science, statistics, mathematics, and other relevant fields into the curriculum to provide a comprehensive understanding.

Case Studies and Examples: To make the content more relatable and applicable to healthcare settings, incorporating real-world case studies and examples demonstrating AI applications in healthcare can enhance learning outcomes.

Benefits and Limitations: It's important to set realistic expectations. The training should highlight the potential of AI in improving healthcare efficiency, diagnosis, and treatment planning. However, it should also address limitations, such as the need for human oversight and the potential for bias in algorithms.

2. Clinical Applications: Provide specialized training modules focusing on the practical applications of AI in various healthcare domains, such as diagnostics, treatment planning, and predictive analytics. Here's a breakdown of what this component should cover:

Domain-Specific Focus: This training moves beyond general concepts and focuses on how AI is being used in specific healthcare areas such as radiology, pathology, cardiology, oncology, and genomics, among others. Examples include:

Diagnostics: Explore AI's role in analysing medical images (X-rays, mammograms) to identify abnormalities, assisting with automated analysis of lab tests, and supporting early disease detection.

Treatment Planning: Discuss how AI can help personalize treatment plans by analysing patient data and suggesting tailored medication regimens or therapies based on historical data and successful cases.

Predictive Analytics: Examine how AI algorithms can analyse vast datasets to predict patient risk factors for specific diseases, allowing for preventative measures or early interventions.

Real-world Examples: Showcase real-world applications of AI in healthcare settings. This could involve case studies, demonstrations of AI-powered software tools, or guest lectures from healthcare professionals already utilizing AI.

Workflow Integration: Discuss how AI can be integrated into existing clinical workflows. This might involve training on utilizing AI tools for data analysis, interpreting AI-generated insights, and effectively communicating findings to patients.

Benefits and Challenges: Analyse the specific benefits and challenges associated with AI in each domain. For example, highlight how AI can improve diagnostic accuracy while acknowledging the need for human expertise in confirming findings.

3. Hands-on Experience: Facilitate hands-on training opportunities, including workshops and simulation exercises, where healthcare professionals can interact with AI tools and algorithms in a controlled environment. Here's what this hands-on experience could look like:

Interactive Workshops: Facilitate workshops where participants can engage with AI platforms or software designed for healthcare applications. This could involve practicing data analysis with AI tools, interpreting AI-generated reports, or simulating the use of AI for decision support in specific scenarios.

Simulation Exercises: Develop interactive simulations that mimic real-world situations where healthcare professionals might encounter AI. This could involve analysing patient data sets with AI support to suggest diagnoses or exploring how AI can be used to personalize treatment plans for virtual patients.

Sandbox Environments: Provide access to "sandbox" environments where healthcare professionals can experiment with AI tools without risk to real patient data. This allows them to explore functionalities, test different approaches with sample datasets, and gain comfort using AI before integrating it into their practice.

Case Studies with Interactive Elements: Present real-world case studies where AI has been used in healthcare. Instead of just reading about it, incorporate interactive elements where participants can analyse the data, make decisions based on AI insights, and explore different scenarios to understand the impact of AI on the decision-making process.

Access to Resources: Offering access to resources such as AI development kits, open-source software libraries, and online tutorials empowers healthcare professionals to continue learning and experimenting with AI beyond formal training sessions.

Guidance from Experts: Having experienced instructors or mentors available to guide participants through hands-on activities ensures that they receive expert guidance and support, enhancing their confidence and competence in using AI technologies.

4. Ethical and Regulatory Considerations: Incorporate modules addressing the ethical, legal, and regulatory aspects of AI in healthcare, emphasizing principles of patient privacy, data security, and algorithm transparency.

Ethical Frameworks: Introduce ethical frameworks for using AI in healthcare, such as principles of fairness, accountability, and patient autonomy. This helps guide healthcare professionals in making responsible decisions about AI use in different scenarios.

Patient Privacy and Data Security: Emphasizing the importance of protecting patient privacy and ensuring data security is essential. Healthcare professionals must understand how AI algorithms handle sensitive patient information and comply with regulations prevail in various countries.

Transparency and Explainability: Healthcare professionals need to understand how AI algorithms arrive at their conclusions. This section should delve into the concept of explainable AI (XAI) and how it can make the decision-making process of AI algorithms more transparent and trustworthy for both healthcare professionals and patients.

Algorithmic Bias: Discuss the potential for bias in AI algorithms, how it can arise from training data, and how it can lead to unfair or discriminatory outcomes in healthcare. Explore strategies to mitigate bias, such as using diverse datasets and ongoing monitoring of algorithms for fairness.

Legal and Regulatory Compliance: Healthcare professionals must be aware of relevant laws, regulations, and guidelines governing the use of AI in healthcare, such as FDA (Food and Drug Administration) regulations for medical devices and software, as well as professional codes of conduct.

5. Lifelong Learning: Foster a culture of lifelong learning by offering ongoing professional development opportunities, including webinars, conferences, and online courses; to keep healthcare professionals abreast of the latest advancements in AI.

Continuous Professional Development: Encouraging healthcare professionals to engage in lifelong learning is essential for staying updated on advancements in AI technology and its applications in healthcare. This involves participating in ongoing training, education, and professional development activities throughout their careers.

Webinars and Conferences: Hosting webinars, seminars, and conferences focused on AI in healthcare allows professionals to stay abreast of the latest research findings, case studies, and best practices. These events provide opportunities for networking, knowledge sharing, and collaboration with peers and experts in the field.

Online Courses and Resources: Offering online courses, self-paced modules, and educational resources on AI and healthcare enables professionals to access learning materials conveniently from anywhere at any time. Platforms such as MOOCs (Massive Open Online Courses) and learning management systems can facilitate continuous learning.

Community Engagement: Establishing communities of practice or professional networks dedicated to AI in healthcare facilitates peer learning, knowledge exchange, and collabouration. These communities provide forums for discussing challenges, sharing experiences, and seeking advice from peers and mentors.

Specialized Certifications: Pursuing specialized certifications or credentials in AI and healthcare demonstrates a commitment to professional development and enhances credibility in the field. Certifying bodies can develop competency frameworks and assessment criteria to ensure that certified professionals possess the necessary knowledge and skills.

Research and Innovation: Encouraging healthcare professionals to engage in research projects, quality improvement initiatives, or innovation challenges related to AI in healthcare fosters a culture of continuous learning and drives advancements in the field. Research findings can contribute to evidence-based practice and inform future training initiatives.

8.3 Collaborations between Healthcare Professionals and AI Experts

Collaboration between healthcare professionals and AI experts is instrumental in driving innovation and maximizing the potential of AI in healthcare. Key strategies for fostering collaboration and benefits include:

1. Interdisciplinary Teams: Form interdisciplinary teams comprising healthcare professionals, data scientists, computer engineers, and other AI experts to leverage diverse perspectives and expertise.
2. Co-creation Initiatives: Engage healthcare professionals in co-creation initiatives where they collaborate with AI experts to design and develop AI solutions tailored to their specific clinical needs and workflows.
3. Knowledge Sharing Platforms: Establish forums, such as conferences, seminars, and online communities, where healthcare professionals and AI experts can exchange knowledge, share best practices, and collaborate on research projects.
4. Mentorship programs: Facilitate mentorship programs that pair healthcare professionals with AI experts, enabling knowledge transfer and skills development in both directions.
5. Research Collaborations: Encourage collaborative research projects that bridge the gap between clinical practice and AI research, fostering innovation and advancing the evidence base for AI applications in healthcare.

Benefits:

Bridging the Knowledge Gap: Healthcare professionals possess deep clinical expertise, but may lack in-depth knowledge of AI algorithms and functionalities. Conversely, AI experts understand the technical intricacies of AI but may not grasp the nuances of medical decision-making. Collaboration bridges this gap, allowing for a synergy of knowledge that fosters effective AI applications in healthcare settings.

Ensuring Ethical Use: AI algorithms can be susceptible to bias, raising ethical concerns. Collaboration between healthcare professionals and AI experts is vital to ensure algorithms are trained on diverse datasets, mitigating bias and promoting fairness in AI-driven healthcare solutions.

Optimizing for Real-World Needs: AI experts can develop powerful algorithms, but healthcare professionals understand the practical realities of clinical workflows and patient interaction. Collaboration ensures that AI tools are designed to seamlessly integrate into existing workflows, optimizing their use for real-world healthcare scenarios.

Building Trust and Transparency: For AI to be widely adopted in healthcare, trust from both patients and healthcare professionals is paramount. Collaboration fosters transparency, allowing healthcare professionals to understand how AI arrives at conclusions and explain them to patients, building trust in AI-assisted decisions.

8.4 Patient Awareness and Education on AI in Healthcare

Patient awareness and education are fundamental to fostering trust and acceptance of AI in healthcare. Key strategies include:

1. Transparent Communication: Provide clear, accessible information about AI technologies, their applications in healthcare, and potential benefits and risks. Use layman's terms and avoid technical jargon to ensure comprehension.

2. Educational Resources: Develop patient-friendly educational materials, such as brochures, videos, and websites, explaining how AI is used in diagnosis, treatment, and preventive care. These resources should emphasize the role of AI as a tool to enhance, not replace, human expertise and judgment.

3. Patient Advocacy Groups: Partner with patient advocacy organizations to disseminate information about AI in healthcare and address patient concerns. These groups can serve as valuable conduits for communication and feedback between patients and healthcare providers.

4. Interactive Workshops: Conduct interactive workshops or seminars where patients can learn about AI first-hand, ask questions, and engage in discussions with healthcare professionals and AI experts.

5. Digital Health Literacy: Enhance patients' digital health literacy by teaching them how to critically evaluate AI-driven health information, navigate digital health platforms, and make informed decisions about their care.

8.5 Patient Engagement in AI-Driven Medical Decisions

Empowering patients to actively participate in AI-driven medical decisions promotes shared

Decision-making and patient-centred care. Strategies to facilitate patient engagement include:

1. Shared Decision-Making Tools: Provide patients with decision aids and interactive tools that leverage AI to present personalized treatment options, risks, and benefits based on individual preferences and clinical data.
2. Informed Consent: Ensure patients understand how AI technologies will be used in their care and obtain their informed consent before implementing AI-driven interventions. Encourage

patients to ask questions and express their preferences and concerns.

3. Personal Health Records: Enable patients to access and contribute to their electronic health records, including AI-generated insights and recommendations. Empowering patients to review and update their health information fosters collaboration and accountability in healthcare decision-making.
4. Patient Decision Support: Offer decision support resources, such as decision trees, patient testimonials, and peer support networks, to help patients navigate complex medical decisions involving AI technologies.
5. Continuous Feedback Loop: Establish mechanisms for patients to provide feedback on their experiences with AI-driven healthcare interventions, including satisfaction, usability, and perceived impact on outcomes. Use this feedback to iterate and improve AI algorithms and clinical protocols.

8.6 Addressing Concerns and Building Trust

Addressing patient concerns and building trust are essential for the successful adoption of AI in healthcare. Strategies to build trust include:

1. Transparency: Be transparent about how AI algorithms are developed, validated, and deployed in clinical practice. Disclose potential biases, limitations, and uncertainties associated with AI technologies to build trust and credibility.
2. Privacy and Data Security: Ensure robust safeguards for patient privacy and data security throughout the AI lifecycle, from data collection and processing to storage and sharing. Adhere to ethical standards and regulatory requirements to protect patient confidentiality and trust.
3. Explainable AI: Prioritize the development of explainable AI models that provide transparent explanations of decision-making processes and recommendations to patients and healthcare

providers. Enhancing transparency and interpretability fosters trust and acceptance of AI-driven healthcare interventions.

4. Cultural Competence: Recognize and respect patients' diverse cultural backgrounds, beliefs, and preferences when integrating AI into healthcare delivery. Culturally competent care enhances patient trust and engagement in AI-driven medical decisions.
5. Patient-Centred Care: Prioritize patient-centred care by soliciting input from patients and involving them as partners in the design, implementation, and evaluation of AI-driven healthcare interventions. Empowering patients as active participants promotes trust, autonomy, and satisfaction in their care.

Chapter
09

DATA IN HEALTHCARE

The importance of data in training AI models cannot be overstated. Data serves as the foundation upon which machine learning algorithms build patterns, make predictions, and generate insights. The quality, quantity, and diversity of the data used directly impact the performance and capabilities of AI models.

9.1 Quality of Data

High-quality data is critical for the accuracy and reliability of AI models in healthcare. This includes data that is clean, well-labeled, and representative of the population. High-quality data helps to reduce biases, minimize errors, and improve the generalizability of the models. For instance, accurate patient records, precise imaging data, and detailed medical histories contribute to better diagnostic tools and treatment plans.

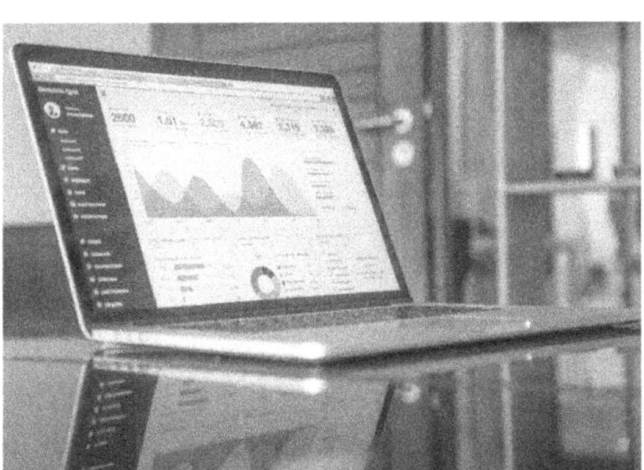

Many ML practitioners often assume that using "Big Data" can compensate for poor data quality. However, this is a misconception. In reality, data quality issues in large datasets can exacerbate problems and lead to worse outcomes for ML models. A simple model trained on high-quality data will consistently outperform a complex model trained on "Big Data" of questionable quality.

The concept of "Garbage in, garbage out" (GIGO) in computing and artificial intelligence underscores the importance of input data quality. It suggests that if the data provided to a system—such as an AI model or algorithm—is of poor quality, inaccurate, or irrelevant, the output will be similarly flawed. AI models, including those in machine learning and deep learning, are heavily reliant on the data used for training and validation. Consequently, if the training data is biased, incomplete, or contains errors, the AI model is likely to produce unreliable or biased results.

9.1.1 Key components of quality data in AI

1. Accuracy: Accurate data is essential for AI algorithms to generate correct and reliable results. When data is precise and error-free, the AI models can make sound decisions and provide insights that are trustworthy. Inaccurate data, on the other hand, can lead to flawed outcomes, potentially causing harm to individuals or organizations.
2. Consistency: Consistency refers to the uniformity of data in terms of format and structure across the dataset. Consistent data allows for seamless processing and analysis, reducing the likelihood of errors during model training. Inconsistent data, however, can lead to confusion, misinterpretation, and a decrease in AI system performance.
3. Completeness: Completeness ensures that all necessary data is present within the dataset. Incomplete data can cause AI algorithms to overlook important patterns or correlations, leading to biased or partial results. Comprehensive data is critical for training AI models effectively, allowing them to learn from the full range of available information.
4. Timeliness: Timeliness refers to the relevance of data in terms of its currency. Data that is up-to-date is vital for AI systems to

accurately reflect current trends, environments, and situations. Outdated data can lead to irrelevant or misleading outputs, as the AI model may base its decisions on information that no longer holds true.

5. Relevance: Relevance means that the data directly pertains to the problem being addressed. Relevant data helps AI systems focus on the most critical variables and relationships, improving the efficiency and accuracy of the model. Irrelevant data, in contrast, can clutter the model, leading to inefficiencies and a dilution of the model's effectiveness.

9.1.2 Challenges of ensuring data quality in AI

1. Data collection: Organizations face the challenge of gathering data from multiple sources while maintaining high quality. Ensuring that all data points adhere to consistent standards and eliminating duplicate or conflicting information is a complex task.
2. Data labelling: Incorrectly labelled data can mislead AI models during training, resulting in poor model performance and unreliable outputs.
3. Data Accessibility and Availability: Ensuring that data is accessible and available for analysis while maintaining its quality can be challenging, especially when dealing with proprietary or restricted data sources.
4. Scalability Issues: As data volumes grow, maintaining data quality at scale becomes increasingly difficult. Large datasets can introduce complexities in processing, storage, and quality control.
5. Data storage and security: Preserving data quality also involves safeguarding it from unauthorized access and potential corruption. Ensuring secure and reliable data storage is essential for organizations.
6. Data governance: This involves coordinating multiple stakeholders, standardizing data practices, and overcoming issues like data silos, inconsistent data formats, and ensuring

compliance with regulatory requirements. Without effective data governance, organizations risk data inaccuracies, inefficiencies, and vulnerabilities to data breaches.

9.1.3 Best practices for ensuring data quality in AI

1. Establish Clear Data Governance: Implement a robust data governance framework to standardize data management practices, enforce quality standards, and ensure accountability across the organization.
2. Data Cleaning and Preprocessing: Regularly clean and preprocess data to remove errors, inconsistencies, duplicates, and irrelevant information before feeding it into AI models. Data quality tools can be used to automate data cleansing, validation, and monitoring processes
3. Continuous Monitoring and Validation: Monitor data quality continuously through automated checks and validation processes to detect and address issues early in the data pipeline.
4. Ensure Data Consistency: Standardize data formats, naming conventions, and structures across all sources to maintain consistency and reduce the risk of misinterpretation.
5. Implement Data Provenance Tracking: Keep track of data origins and transformations to maintain transparency, traceability, and accountability, which is essential for ensuring the integrity of the data.
6. Regularly Update Data: Keep datasets current by regularly updating them to reflect the most recent trends, conditions, and changes in the environment.
7. Incorporate Data Auditing: Perform regular audits to review data quality, identify any issues, and make necessary corrections to maintain high standards.
8. Educate and Train Teams: Ensure that all team members involved in data management and AI development understand the importance of data quality and are trained in best practices to maintain it.

9.2 Quantity of Data

The quantity of data available for training AI models is crucial to their performance, as data is essentially the lifeblood of any machine learning project. However, determining the exact amount of data required isn't straightforward—there isn't a universal answer to the question of how much data is needed for machine learning. Large datasets allow models to learn intricate patterns, enhancing their predictive accuracy.

One commonly used guideline is the "10 times rule," which suggests that the number of data samples should be at least ten times greater than the number of parameters or degrees of freedom in the model. For instance, if a model differentiates between images of cats and dogs using 1,000 parameters, it would typically require around 10,000 images to train effectively. While this rule is useful for smaller models, it doesn't always hold true for larger, more complex models. In these cases, the number of examples doesn't necessarily correlate with the actual amount of data required for training.

In the healthcare sector, having access to extensive patient data—such as electronic health records (EHRs), medical images, and genomic information—is essential for developing robust AI solutions. These models can be utilized to predict disease outbreaks, tailor treatment plans to individual patients, and ultimately improve patient outcomes.

9.2.1 Data Adequacy

The amount of data required to train a machine learning model depends on several factors

1. Model Complexity

Simple Models: Models like linear regression or decision trees generally require less data because they have fewer parameters to learn.

Complex Models: Deep learning models, especially deep neural networks with many layers and parameters, require significantly more data to avoid overfitting and to capture the underlying patterns.

2. Dimensionality of Data

Low-Dimensional Data: If the data has fewer features (e.g., 2-3 features), fewer examples may be sufficient for the model to learn effectively.

High-Dimensional Data: In cases where the data has many features (e.g., image data with thousands of pixels), more data is typically needed to ensure that the model can learn the relationships between features without overfitting.

3. Variability in Data

High Variability: If the data is highly diverse (e.g., many different classes in classification or a wide range of values in regression), more data is needed to ensure that all variations are adequately captured.

Low Variability: For data with less variability, fewer examples might be sufficient.

4. Class Imbalance

Balanced Classes: If the classes in the dataset are balanced, the model can learn effectively with a moderate amount of data.

Imbalanced Classes: If one class is significantly underrepresented, more data (especially for the minority class) may be needed to train a model that performs well across all classes.

5. Noise in Data

Noisy Data: If the data contains a lot of noise (irrelevant or random information), more data might be required to help the model learn the underlying patterns and avoid fitting the noise.

Clean Data: Clean, well-curated data requires less data overall because the model doesn't have to filter out as much noise.

6. Overfitting Concerns

Risk of Overfitting: To prevent overfitting, especially in complex models, a larger dataset is typically required. This allows the model to generalize better to new, unseen data.

Regularization: Techniques like regularization can help reduce the amount of data needed, but they may not completely eliminate the need for more data in complex scenarios.

7. Domain-Specific Requirements

Domain Knowledge: In some domains (e.g., medical imaging), even small datasets can be sufficient if they are highly curated and each example is rich in information. In other domains, large datasets are necessary to capture the full scope of the problem.

General Guidelines:

Rule of Thumb: For many applications, hundreds to thousands of examples per class or category are often needed for basic models, while deep learning models may require tens of thousands or more.

Empirical Testing: Often, the exact amount of data needed is determined through experimentation. Start with a smaller dataset, train the model, and observe its performance. Gradually increase the dataset size and monitor improvements.

9.2.2 Tips to reduce data need for ML

While larger datasets often lead to better results, they aren't always necessary. Here are some practical strategies to reduce the amount of data needed for machine learning:

- Pre-trained Models: Enhance your machine learning model with pre-trained models, which bring pre-existing knowledge. For instance, models like ResNet for image recognition or BERT for natural language processing can be fine-tuned on your specific task using a smaller dataset. This approach allows you to build a powerful model without needing vast amounts of initial training data.
- Transfer Learning: Transfer learning reduces the quantity of required data by leveraging a model pretrained on a large dataset

in a related domain. Suppose you've trained a model to recognize cats in images and now want it to detect dogs. Instead of starting from scratch, you can use transfer learning. This technique allows you to leverage the features learned from the cat recognition task and adapt them to identify dogs, requiring only a smaller dataset of dog images. This "knowledge transfer" saves time, resources, and data.

- Feature Engineering: Not all data points are equally important. Identify and use only the most important features that contribute to the model's predictions. This reduces the dimensionality of the problem, often lowering the data requirement.
- Data Augmentation: Expand your dataset by using techniques such as image flipping, text synonym replacement, or generating synthetic data points. This increased diversity helps your machine learning model generalize better and perform well, even with limited original data.
- Experiment with Combinations: Experimentation is key to enhancing your results. Try different combinations of these techniques to see what works best for your specific task and dataset. More complex models may require experimenting with more sophisticated combinations as well.

A 2020 Kaggle survey revealed that 70% of respondents had completed a machine learning project with fewer than 10,000 samples, and over half had completed a project with fewer than 5,000 samples. At Stanford University, a team used just 1,000 images to develop an AI system capable of diagnosing skin cancer. Similarly, a team at MIT created an AI system to detect diabetic retinopathy in eye scans using only 500 images.

9.3 Diversity of Data

Seeking a second opinion is a common practice among humans, and the same principle applies to automation employing machine learning.

Industry experts have noted a growing emphasis on data that provides a more comprehensive situational analysis, often referred to as a "360-degree view." To distinguish this from "big data," they coined the term "wide data" a few years ago. The need for data diversity is essential, particularly in healthcare, where patient populations are highly diverse. Diverse datasets expose AI models to a broader range of scenarios and conditions, making them more inclusive and effective across different demographics, such as age, gender, ethnicity, and socio-economic status. For instance, a model trained on a diverse dataset is better equipped to identify and treat diseases in various populations, helping to reduce health disparities.

9.3.1 Benefit of Data Diversity

Improved Generalization: Diverse training data helps AI models generalize better to new, unseen data. When models are trained on a wide range of examples from different demographics, regions, and scenarios, they can learn more comprehensive patterns and features. This reduces the risk of overfitting to specific subsets of data and enhances the model's ability to make accurate predictions in real-world situations.

Reduced Bias: Homogeneous datasets can introduce biases that skew AI predictions and decisions. These biases may be related to ethnicity, gender, location or other factors. By including diverse data, AI developers can identify and mitigate biases more effectively. Diverse datasets provide a broader perspective on different groups and scenarios, helping to create more fair and equitable AI systems.

Enhanced Robustness: AI models trained on diverse datasets are more robust against variations and changes in data distribution. They are better equipped to handle edge cases and outliers that may not be well-represented in more homogeneous datasets. This robustness is essential for deploying AI systems in dynamic environments where data can vary widely.

Real-World Applicability: AI systems are designed to solve real-world problems and interact with diverse populations. Training them on diverse datasets ensures that they can handle the complexities and nuances present in the real world. This leads to more practical and effective AI solutions that can address a wide range of challenges across various domains.

Innovation and Adaptation: Diverse training data encourages innovation in AI research and development. It opens up new possibilities for exploring different data types, modalities, and sources, which can lead to breakthroughs in AI capabilities. This diversity fosters creativity and encourages the development of AI systems that can adapt to evolving data landscapes and user needs.

Handling edge use cases: Diverse training data incorporates examples from various scenarios, including rare and edge cases. This exposure enables the model to learn how to manage challenging situations that might be underrepresented in the data but are still likely to occur in real-world applications.

Ethical Considerations: Ensuring diversity in training data is crucial from an ethical standpoint. It promotes fairness and inclusivity in AI applications by ensuring that all individuals, regardless of their background or characteristics, are represented fairly in the decision-making processes of AI systems. This helps in building trust and acceptance of AI technologies among diverse user groups

9.3.2 How to ensure Diversity in Training Data?

Define Diversity Goals: Clearly define what diversity means in the context of your AI application. Consider demographic factors (such as age, gender, ethnicity), geographic diversity, socioeconomic status, and other relevant characteristics based on the application domain.

Curate Representative Datasets: Start by curating datasets that are representative of the population or problem space your AI system will encounter. Ensure that the dataset includes examples from diverse demographics, regions, and scenarios that are relevant to your application.

Data Collection Strategies: Employ diverse data collection strategies to gather data from various sources and populations. This may involve partnerships with diverse communities, organizations, or using data collection methods that capture a wide range of perspectives and experiences.

Data Augmentation: Use data augmentation techniques to increase the diversity within your existing dataset. This could include techniques such as synthesizing additional examples, translating text into different languages, or altering images to represent different demographics.

Balancing Data Representation: Ensure that each subgroup within your dataset is adequately represented to avoid biases. Use stratified sampling techniques to maintain proportional representation of different groups, especially when datasets are imbalanced.

Regularly evaluate and Update: Continuously monitor and evaluate the diversity of your training data. As new data becomes available or as your AI system evolves, update the dataset to reflect changing demographics and contexts.

Mitigate Bias: Be mindful of biases that may exist within your data collection process or dataset. Implement techniques such as bias detection algorithms, fairness metrics, and bias mitigation strategies to address and mitigate biases that could impact AI model performance.

Identify Rare and Edge Cases: Start by identifying what constitutes rare and edge cases relevant to your AI application. These could be scenarios that are uncommon but still impactful, outliers, or situations where standard models might struggle.

Collaborate and Share: Collaborate with diverse stakeholders, researchers, and communities to enrich your understanding of the diversity landscape relevant to your AI application. Share insights and collaborate on initiatives to improve diversity in AI datasets collectively.

Educate and Train: Educate AI practitioners and data scientists about the importance of diversity in training data and provide training on best practices for achieving diversity. Foster a culture of diversity and inclusion within AI development teams.

9.4 The Role of Data in Training AI Models

1. Learning Patterns and Representations: AI models, especially those based on machine learning; learn from patterns present in data. The more diverse and representative the data, the better the model can capture complex relationships and make accurate predictions. Quality data is essential for the model to generalize well to new, unseen instances.
2. Model Training and Optimization: During the training phase, AI models adjust their parameters based on the input data to minimize the difference between predicted outputs and actual outcomes. The training process involves exposing the model to a variety of data, enabling it to learn the underlying patterns and relationships present in the information.
3. Feature Extraction and Representation Learning: Features are the characteristics or attributes extracted from the data that influence the model's decision-making. Effective feature extraction is crucial for representing the relevant information in the dataset. Well-curated and diverse datasets help the model learn informative features, contributing to better performance.
4. Generalization and Adaptability: The ability of an AI model to generalize to new, unseen data depends on the diversity and representativeness of the training data. If the model is trained on a narrow or biased dataset, it may struggle to perform well on real-world scenarios with variations in data distribution.
5. Reducing Bias and Fairness: Biases present in training data can be inherited by AI models. It is crucial to carefully curate datasets to mitigate biases and ensure fairness in predictions. Understanding

and addressing biases in data contribute to the ethical development and deployment of AI models.

6. Supervised Learning Labels: In supervised learning, where the model is trained on labeled data, the accuracy and relevance of labels significantly impact the model's performance. High-quality labeled datasets are essential for teaching the model to associate input features with correct outputs.
7. Unsupervised Learning and Clustering: Unsupervised learning models, such as clustering algorithms, rely on patterns and structures within the data. These models uncover hidden relationships without labelled examples. Comprehensive and diverse datasets assist in revealing meaningful patterns and groupings.
8. Transfer Learning and Pre-trained Models: Transfer learning involves using a pre-trained model on a large dataset for a specific task before fine-tuning it for a new task with a smaller dataset. The success of transfer learning hinges on the quality and representativeness of the initial pre-training data.
9. Robustness and Resilience: Robust AI models that perform well under various conditions and against adversarial attacks are trained on diverse datasets. Ensuring that the training data includes a wide range of scenarios helps the model become more resilient to unexpected inputs.
10. Real-World Applicability: The ultimate goal of AI is to perform well in real-world scenarios. A diverse and well-curated dataset ensures that the AI model is equipped to handle the complexities, variations, and challenges present in the target application or environment.

In summary, data serves as the lifeblood of AI model training, influencing their accuracy, reliability, and generalization capabilities. Thorough consideration of data quality, diversity, and representativeness is essential for developing effective and responsible AI systems. Continuous monitoring and updating of datasets contribute to the ongoing improvement of AI models over time.

9.4.1 Role of Data-A Healthcare Perspective

In the realm of healthcare, the importance of data in training AI models is paramount, as it directly impacts the efficacy, accuracy, and ethical considerations of these systems. The healthcare sector is undergoing a transformative shift with the integration of artificial intelligence, and the quality of data utilized plays a pivotal role in shaping the success and reliability of AI models in this context.

1. Patient-Centric Care: Healthcare AI models aim to provide patient-centric care by leveraging data to understand individual health profiles, medical histories, and treatment responses. Comprehensive and diverse datasets ensure that the AI systems can generate personalized insights, leading to more effective diagnosis, treatment plans, and patient outcomes.
2. Clinical Decision Support: AI models in healthcare act as powerful clinical decision support tools for healthcare professionals. The accuracy of these decision-making systems relies heavily on the quality and breadth of the data used for training. Well-curated datasets contribute to the model's ability to analyse complex medical scenarios and provide evidence-based recommendations.
3. Disease Prediction and Prevention: The use of AI for predicting disease susceptibility and preventing the onset of illnesses is contingent on access to extensive and representative health data. Robust datasets enable machine learning algorithms to identify subtle patterns, risk factors, and early indicators, facilitating proactive interventions and preventive healthcare measures.
4. Diagnostic Accuracy: AI models play a crucial role in medical imaging, aiding in the interpretation of radiological images for diagnosis. Training these models requires high-quality datasets that encompass a wide variety of imaging modalities and clinical conditions. Accurate and diverse data contribute to the model's ability to detect abnormalities and assist healthcare professionals in making more precise diagnoses.

5. Drug Discovery and Development: In pharmaceutical research, AI models analyse vast datasets to expedite drug discovery and development processes. Comprehensive datasets, including molecular structures, genetic information, and clinical trial outcomes, are essential for training models that can predict drug efficacy, safety, and potential side effects.
6. Population Health Management: AI models in healthcare are utilized for population health management, requiring data that reflects the diversity of populations and their health dynamics. These models can identify trends, assess risk factors, and allocate resources efficiently based on the analysis of large and varied datasets.
7. Ethical Considerations and Bias Mitigation: The ethical use of AI in healthcare demands careful consideration of biases present in training data. Biased datasets can lead to disparities in healthcare outcomes. Therefore, efforts to curate unbiased and representative datasets are essential to ensure fair and equitable AI applications in healthcare.

In conclusion, data is the cornerstone of AI model development in healthcare, influencing every aspect of patient care, diagnosis, treatment, and research. The responsible and effective integration of AI in healthcare necessitates a concerted effort to curate, manage, and leverage high-quality datasets, ensuring that AI technologies contribute positively to the advancement of healthcare outcomes while maintaining the highest standards of patient privacy and ethical considerations.

9.5 Data Sources in Healthcare AI

In healthcare AI, data sources are crucial for developing accurate models and deriving meaningful insights. Here are some key sources of data in this domain:

9.5.1 Electronic Health Records (EHRs)

Today, the medical field has transitioned from traditional paper-based records to digital systems for storing information, specifically through Electronic Health Records (EHR). An Electronic Health Record (EHR) is a digital version of a patient's medical history, which is maintained by the healthcare provider over time. This record may encompass all essential administrative and clinical data pertinent to a person's care under a specific provider, including medical issues, progress notes, medications, laboratory results, radiology reports, vital signs, demographics, past medical history, and immunizations.

EHRs enhance the accessibility of information, offering the potential to streamline the clinician's workflow. Additionally, EHRs can support various care-related activities, either directly or indirectly, through different interfaces. These include evidence-based decision support, quality management, and outcomes reporting. Here's a detailed exploration of EHRs:

1. Comprehensive Patient Information: EHRs consolidate patient information from various sources such as medical history, medications, allergies, immunizations, lab results, diagnostic images, and progress notes. This holistic view enables healthcare providers to make informed decisions quickly and efficiently, enhancing the quality of patient care.
2. Accessibility and Interoperability: Unlike paper records, EHRs facilitate seamless sharing of information among healthcare providers within the same organization or across different healthcare settings (e.g., hospitals, clinics, pharmacies). This interoperability improves care coordination, reduces duplication of tests, and enhances patient safety.
3. Efficiency and Workflow Improvement: EHRs streamline administrative tasks by automating processes such as appointment scheduling, billing, and prescription ordering. Clinicians can electronically prescribe medications, reducing errors associated

with handwriting and improving medication adherence monitoring.

4. Decision Support and Clinical Guidance: EHR systems often include clinical decision support tools that provide alerts for drug interactions, reminders for preventive care screenings, evidence-based treatment guidelines, and personalized recommendations based on patient data. These tools assist healthcare providers in delivering more effective and personalized care.
5. Patient Engagement and Empowerment: Patients can access their EHRs through secure portals, allowing them to review their medical history, lab results, appointment schedules, and communicate with their healthcare team. This transparency fosters patient engagement, encourages shared decision-making, and improves health literacy.
6. Data Analytics and Population Health Management: EHRs support population health management initiatives by aggregating anonymized patient data for analysis. Healthcare organizations can identify trends, monitor disease outbreaks, track patient outcomes, and implement targeted interventions to improve public health.
7. Regulatory Compliance and Security: EHR systems adhere to stringent regulatory standards to protect patient privacy and confidentiality. They employ robust security measures such as encryption, authentication controls, and audit trails to safeguard sensitive health information from unauthorized access or breaches.

9.5.1. a. Challenges of EHR

Electronic Health Records (EHRs) offer significant advantages in healthcare, but they also come with several challenges that impact their implementation, adoption, and use. Here are some key challenges associated with EHRs:

1. Cost of Implementation and Maintenance: Implementing an EHR system involves significant upfront costs, including software

purchase, hardware infrastructure, training, and customization. Ongoing maintenance, upgrades, and support also incur additional expenses.

2. Interoperability Issues: EHR systems often face challenges in exchanging data seamlessly with other systems, both within the same healthcare organization and across different healthcare settings. Incompatible formats, standards, and protocols hinder the efficient sharing of patient information.
3. User Interface and Usability Concerns: Poorly designed user interfaces and complex workflows can lead to usability issues for healthcare providers. Data entry processes may be time-consuming and cumbersome, potentially impacting clinical productivity and user satisfaction.
4. Data Security and Privacy Risks: EHRs store sensitive patient information, making them attractive targets for cyberattacks and data breaches. Ensuring robust security measures (e.g., encryption, access controls) and complying with privacy regulations are critical but challenging tasks.
5. Workflow Disruptions and Training Needs: Transitioning from paper-based records to EHRs can disrupt established workflows within healthcare organizations. Adequate training and support for healthcare providers and staff are essential to minimize productivity losses and ensure effective system utilization.
6. Data Accuracy and Integrity: EHRs rely on accurate and complete data entry by healthcare providers. Errors in data entry, duplicate records, and inconsistencies in documentation can compromise the quality and reliability of patient information, affecting clinical decision-making.
7. Resistance to Change and Cultural Shifts: Some healthcare professionals may resist adopting EHRs due to concerns about changes in clinical practices, perceived loss of autonomy, or unfamiliarity with technology. Overcoming resistance requires effective change management strategies and ongoing support.

8. Regulatory Compliance Challenges: EHR systems must comply with regulatory requirements and standards related to patient privacy, data security, and interoperability. Staying abreast of evolving regulations and implementing necessary updates can be complex and resource-intensive.
9. Integration with Other Technologies: Integrating EHRs with other healthcare technologies (e.g., medical devices, telehealth platforms) to support coordinated care and data exchange poses technical challenges. Ensuring seamless integration and interoperability remains a priority for healthcare IT teams.
10. Impact on Patient-Provider Relationship: The use of EHRs during patient consultations may potentially affect the patient-provider interaction, with concerns about reduced face-to-face interaction and perceived distractions from computer screens.

9.5.1. b. Types of EHR

1. Electronic Health Records (EHRs) come in various types, catering to different healthcare needs and settings. Here are some common types:
2. Standalone EHRs: These systems operate independently within a single healthcare facility. They do not communicate with other EHR systems outside the organization. Ideal for small practices or individual clinics.
3. Integrated EHRs: These systems are designed to integrate with other systems within a healthcare organization, such as billing systems, practice management software, and lab systems. They offer a more seamless workflow within a single organization.
4. Interoperable EHRs: These EHR systems are capable of sharing information across different healthcare organizations. They adhere to standardized protocols for data exchange, facilitating coordinated care among multiple providers.
5. Web-Based EHRs: These systems are hosted on the internet and accessed through web browsers. They offer flexibility and ease of

access from any location with internet connectivity, making them suitable for practices with multiple locations or remote care.

6. On-Premise EHRs: These systems are installed and run on local servers within the healthcare facility. They offer greater control over data and customization but require significant IT infrastructure and support.
7. Cloud-Based EHRs: Hosted on remote servers and accessed via the internet, cloud-based EHRs reduce the need for extensive local IT infrastructure. They offer scalability, automatic updates, and easier data backup and recovery.
8. Specialty-Specific EHRs: These EHR systems are tailored to meet the unique needs of specific medical specialties, such as pediatrics, oncology, or cardiology. They include specialty-specific templates, workflows, and features.
9. Personal Health Records (PHRs): While not exactly EHRs, PHRs are maintained by patients themselves. They can integrate with EHR systems to allow patients to manage and access their health information.
10. Mobile EHRs: Designed for use on mobile devices such as tablets and smartphones, these EHRs provide healthcare providers with the flexibility to access and update patient records on the go.
11. Open-Source EHRs: These systems have source code that is freely available for modification and distribution. They allow healthcare organizations to customize the software to their specific needs without the constraints of proprietary software.

9.5.2 Medical Imaging

Medical imaging encompasses various technologies designed to visualize the human body, aiding in the diagnosis, monitoring, or treatment of medical conditions. These techniques are primarily non-invasive, allowing medical professionals to detect injuries, diagnose diseases, or manage chronic conditions without the need for invasive procedures.

Medical imaging datasets are pivotal in advancing AI in healthcare, as they offer extensive volumes of labeled data that AI algorithms can utilize for learning. Data from imaging modalities such as X-rays, MRIs, and CT scans are fundamental in developing AI-driven diagnostic tools. Here's how medical imaging datasets contribute to the advancement of AI in healthcare:

1. Training AI Algorithms: Medical imaging datasets serve as the foundation for training AI models, particularly deep learning models. These datasets typically include thousands to millions of annotated images (e.g., X-rays, MRIs, CT scans) that enable algorithms to learn to recognize patterns, structures, and abnormalities indicative of various diseases.
2. Improving Diagnostic Accuracy: AI algorithms trained on diverse medical imaging datasets can achieve high levels of accuracy in detecting and diagnosing diseases. For example, AI can analyse chest X-rays to detect pneumonia or identify subtle changes in brain MRIs that may indicate early stages of Alzheimer's disease.
3. Enabling Early Detection and Prevention: By analyzing historical imaging data, AI can identify patterns and biomarkers that precede clinical symptoms. This capability supports early detection of diseases such as cancer or cardiovascular conditions, potentially leading to earlier intervention and improved patient outcomes.
4. Facilitating Personalized Medicine: Medical imaging datasets allow AI to develop models that predict patient outcomes and response to treatments based on individual characteristics and imaging biomarkers. This facilitates personalized treatment plans tailored to each patient's unique condition and characteristics.
5. Supporting Clinical Decision Making: AI models trained on medical imaging datasets can provide decision support to radiologists and clinicians by highlighting areas of concern, suggesting differential diagnoses, or recommending further diagnostic tests. This assists healthcare providers in making more informed decisions and reduces diagnostic errors.

6. Accelerating Research and Development: Medical imaging datasets are valuable for medical research and development of new diagnostic tools and therapies. AI can analyse large datasets to identify new imaging biomarkers, validate hypotheses, and streamline clinical trials by identifying suitable patient cohorts.
7. Enhancing Workflow Efficiency: AI-powered tools that integrate with medical imaging workflows can automate routine tasks such as image segmentation, annotation, and data retrieval. This enhances workflow efficiency, reduces interpretation times, and allows radiologists to focus on complex cases requiring human expertise.
8. Addressing Healthcare Disparities: Access to large, diverse medical imaging datasets enables AI to address healthcare disparities by improving diagnostic capabilities in underserved or remote regions. Telemedicine platforms equipped with AI can provide expert-level diagnostics remotely, bridging gaps in access to healthcare.

Here's a breakdown of where to find medical image data sources for ML training:

Public Repositories

- Open-source datasets: Several resources offer free, publicly available medical image datasets. Repositories like Kaggle [Search Kaggle medical image datasets] host datasets on chest X-rays, mammograms, and more.
- Consortiums and Research Institutions: Organizations like The Cancer Imaging Archive (TCIA) [Search cancer imaging archive on The Cancer Imaging Archive (.gov) cancerimagingarchive.net] provide datasets across various cancer types.

Considerations for Public Repositories

❖ Data size: Public datasets may not always have the volume needed for complex models.

- ❖ Data quality: Labelling accuracy and consistency can vary across datasets.
- ❖ Data privacy: Public datasets may have limitations on usage due to privacy concerns.

Commercial Vendors:

- Specialized Data Providers: Companies like CapeStart offer high-quality, curated medical image datasets with rich annotations.

Considerations for Commercial Vendors

- ❖ Cost: Accessing these datasets typically involves a subscription fee.
- ❖ Data access: Data may be delivered through secure platforms with restricted download options.

Additional Resources

- re3data: This comprehensive registry [Search re3data medical imaging datasets] curates information on various medical research data repositories, including those with medical imaging datasets.
- Machine Learning Dataset Repositories: Platforms like Papers With Code [Search papers with code medical datasets] list medical image datasets relevant to specific tasks like medical question answering.

Despite the benefits, utilizing medical image data for ML training presents challenges related to data privacy, regulatory compliance, data heterogeneity, and variability in imaging protocols. Addressing these challenges requires robust data governance frameworks, anonymization techniques, and collaborations between healthcare providers, researchers, and regulatory bodies.

ML-trained models on medical image data have demonstrated promising results in various clinical applications. These include automated disease detection (e.g., lung nodules, breast lesions), quantitative image analysis (e.g., tumourvolumetric), treatment response assessment, and predicting patient outcomes based on imaging biomarkers.

9.5.3 Genomic Data

In the realm of healthcare, the integration of genomic data with machine learning (ML) has opened new avenues for personalized medicine, disease prediction, and understanding genetic factors underlying complex conditions. Genomic data, which encompasses information about an individual's DNA sequence and variations, provides a wealth of insights that ML algorithms can leverage to improve patient outcomes and advance biomedical research. Here's how genomic data contributes to ML training and its impact on healthcare:

1. Understanding Genetic Variation: Genomic data includes variations such as single nucleotide polymorphisms (SNPs), insertions, deletions, and structural variants across the genome. ML algorithms trained on genomic datasets can identify patterns and correlations between genetic variations and disease susceptibility, drug response, and predisposition to certain conditions.
2. Personalized Medicine and Treatment Optimization: ML models trained on genomic data can predict how individuals may respond to specific treatments based on their genetic profiles. This capability supports personalized medicine approaches by tailoring treatments to genetic predispositions, minimizing adverse effects, and optimizing therapeutic outcomes.
3. Disease Prediction and Risk Assessment: By analysing large-scale genomic datasets from cohorts of patients with and without specific diseases, ML algorithms can identify genetic markers associated with disease risk. This facilitates early disease detection, risk assessment, and proactive interventions to mitigate risks before symptoms manifest.
4. Integrating Multi-Omics Data: Genomic data is often integrated with other omics data such as transcriptomics, proteomics, and metabolomics. ML techniques enable the integration and analysis of multi-omics datasets to uncover complex biological interactions, biomarkers, and molecular pathways implicated in disease mechanisms.

5. Pharmacogenomics and Drug Development: ML models trained on genomic and pharmacological data can predict how genetic variations influence drug metabolism, efficacy, and toxicity. This knowledge informs precision medicine strategies by guiding drug selection, dosage optimization, and personalized treatment plans tailored to individual genetic profiles.
6. Challenges and Considerations: Challenges in leveraging genomic data for ML training include data privacy concerns, ethical implications of genetic testing, data standardization across different genomic platforms, and the need for robust algorithms capable of handling high-dimensional and heterogeneous data.
7. Advancing Biomedical Research: ML-driven analysis of genomic data accelerates biomedical research by enabling large-scale genome-wide association studies (GWAS), identifying novel disease biomarkers, elucidating gene-disease interactions, and facilitating the discovery of potential therapeutic targets.
8. Future Directions: Future advancements in ML for genomic data are poised to enhance interpretability of genetic findings, improve prediction accuracy for complex diseases with multifactorial etiologies, and enable real-time genomic analysis integrated into clinical decision support systems.

9.5.4 Wearable Devices

Wearable devices have emerged as transformative tools in healthcare, providing continuous monitoring of physiological parameters and lifestyle behaviours in real-time. These devices, equipped with sensors that capture biometric data such as heart rate, activity levels, sleep patterns, and more, generate vast streams of personalized data. Machine learning (ML) algorithms trained on wearable device data are revolutionizing healthcare by enabling early disease detection, personalized interventions, and improved management of chronic conditions. Here's how wearable devices contribute to ML training and their impact on healthcare:

1. Continuous Data Streams for Personalization: Wearable devices capture real-time biometric data, offering a continuous stream of information about an individual's health status and daily activities. ML algorithms trained on these data can detect subtle changes or anomalies in physiological parameters, facilitating early intervention and personalized health recommendations.
2. Predictive Analytics and Disease Prevention: ML models analyse longitudinal data from wearable devices to predict health outcomes, such as predicting episodes of cardiac arrhythmias based on heart rate variability patterns or identifying early signs of diabetes through glucose monitoring. This predictive capability supports proactive disease prevention strategies and reduces healthcare costs associated with reactive treatments.
3. Behaviour Monitoring and Lifestyle Interventions: Beyond physiological metrics, wearable devices track lifestyle behaviours such as physical activity, sleep quality, and dietary habits. ML algorithms can analyse these behavioural data patterns to identify factors influencing health outcomes, personalize lifestyle interventions, and promote healthy behaviour changes.
4. Remote Patient Monitoring and Telemedicine: Wearable devices enable remote patient monitoring, allowing healthcare providers to monitor patients' health status outside traditional clinical settings. ML-powered analytics on wearable data can alert clinicians to potential health emergencies, track treatment adherence, and optimize remote care delivery, especially in underserved or rural areas.
5. Integration with Electronic Health Records (EHRs): Integrating wearable device data with EHRs enriches patient health records with real-time, objective measurements. ML algorithms can fuse wearable data with historical medical records to provide comprehensive insights into patient health trends, support clinical decision-making, and enhance continuity of care.

6. Challenges and Considerations: Challenges in leveraging wearable device data for ML training include ensuring data accuracy, addressing data privacy concerns, managing interoperability with existing healthcare systems, and overcoming variability in device accuracy and reliability. Addressing these challenges requires robust data governance frameworks, standards for data interoperability, and algorithms resilient to noisy sensor data.
7. Advancing Personalized Healthcare: ML-driven insights from wearable device data empower individuals to actively participate in their healthcare management. By providing personalized health recommendations based on real-time data, wearable devices encourage preventive healthcare behaviours, improve patient engagement, and foster a proactive approach to managing chronic conditions.
8. Future Directions: Future advancements in ML for wearable devices are expected to focus on enhancing algorithm robustness for real-time data analysis, integrating multi-modal data from diverse wearable sensors, and developing AI-driven predictive models that adapt to individual health trajectories over time

9.5.5 Clinical Trials

Clinical trials are the backbone of medical progress, meticulously evaluating the safety and efficacy of new drugs and treatments. However, the vast amount of data generated during these trials, including patient demographics, medical history, treatment responses, and side effects, holds tremendous potential beyond traditional analysis. This is where Machine Learning (ML) steps in.

Unlocking Insights with ML:

ML algorithms can analyse vast amounts of clinical trial data, uncovering hidden patterns and relationships that might be missed by traditional statistical methods. Here's how:

- Predictive Modelling: ML can predict patient responses to treatments, allowing for personalized medicine. By analysing factors like genetics and medical history, models can identify patients most likely to benefit from a specific therapy.
- Trial Optimization: ML can streamline clinical trial design by predicting which trials are most likely to succeed. This reduces costs and accelerates the development of life-saving treatments.
- Adverse Event Detection: ML can be used to identify potential side effects earlier in the trial process, improving patient safety.

Challenges and Considerations:

While promising, using clinical trial data for ML training presents challenges:

- Data Privacy: Patient privacy is paramount. Secure data handling and anonymization techniques are crucial to ensure ethical use of data.
- Data Quality: Clinical trial data can be heterogeneous, with inconsistencies in format and collection methods. Data cleaning and standardization are essential before training ML models.
- Regulatory Landscape: Regulations governing the use of patient data for ML applications are still evolving. Understanding and adhering to these regulations is critical.

Accessing Clinical Trial Data:

Several avenues exist for accessing clinical trial data for ML training:

- Public Databases: Resources like [Search ClinicalTrials.gov] provide access to publicly available clinical trial data. However, the data may be limited in scope or detail.
- Data Sharing Platforms: Initiatives like [Search Sage Bionetworks] promote data sharing within the scientific community. This can provide researchers with access to rich datasets with proper consent and oversight.

- Collaboration with Pharmaceutical Companies: Pharmaceutical companies often hold vast datasets from their own trials. Collaboration with these companies can provide access to highly relevant data, but agreements regarding data ownership and usage need to be established.

The integration of ML into clinical trials has the potential to revolutionize how we develop new therapies. As data security and regulatory frameworks evolve, researchers will have access to richer datasets, enabling them to build more robust and impactful ML models, ultimately accelerating the path towards personalized medicine and improved patient outcomes.

Choosing the Right Data Source

The ideal data source depends on your specific needs. Consider factors like:

- Project goal: What disease or condition are you focusing on?
- Model complexity: How much data is needed to train your model effectively?
- Data privacy requirements: Does your project require anonymized data?
- Budgetary constraints:

9.6 Data Types in Healthcare AI

In the realm of healthcare AI, various types of data play crucial roles in training and refining machine learning models. These data types encompass a broad spectrum of information, each contributing uniquely to enhancing patient care, clinical decision-making, and medical research.

Text Data: Text data in healthcare refers to written or typed information related to patient care, medical literature, or patient-reported data. This includes clinical notes, medical literature, and patient-reported information such as symptoms and medical history. The richness of text data allows AI to understand and interpret complex medical narratives and extract valuable insights.

Tabular Data: Tabular data in healthcare refers to structured data organized in rows and columns, typically stored in databases or spreadsheets. This type of data is commonly used for various purposes in healthcare, including patient management, clinical research, and healthcare analytics. Examples include information about patients, such as their names, ages, genders, addresses, contact details, and insurance information. The structured nature of tabular data makes it ideal for statistical analysis and reporting.

Image Data: Image data in healthcare comprises visual representations obtained from diagnostic procedures, pathology slides, or dermatological imaging. Examples include X-rays, CT scans, MRI scans, pathology slides, and images documenting skin conditions. Image data is essential for developing AI models that can assist in the detection, diagnosis, and monitoring of various medical conditions through advanced image recognition and analysis techniques.

Video Data: Video data in healthcare refers to recorded footage of medical procedures, telemedicine consultations, or physical therapy sessions. This includes surgical videos, telehealth appointments, and recordings of therapeutic exercises. Video data provides a dynamic view of medical activities, allowing for real-time analysis and review, which can improve procedural training and patient care.

Audio Data: Audio data in healthcare encompasses recorded sound files containing medical dictations, telehealth calls, or patient testimonials. This includes audio recordings of healthcare providers dictating clinical notes, telehealth appointments, and patient feedback. Audio data can be used to develop AI models that transcribe, analyse, and interpret spoken language, facilitating documentation and enhancing patient-provider communication.

Sensor Data: Sensor data in healthcare consists of information collected from wearable devices or remote patient monitoring systems. This includes data from fitness trackers, smartwatches, glucose monitors, blood pressure cuffs, and other medical-grade sensors capturing vital signs and activity levels. Sensor data enables continuous health monitoring, providing valuable insights into patients' daily activities and physiological conditions.

9.7 Challenges in Healthcare Data Management

Healthcare data management is a complex undertaking that involves handling, storing, and utilizing vast amounts of sensitive information crucial for patient care, research, and administrative processes. However, this process comes with various challenges, ranging from data security concerns to interoperability issues. This section delves into some of the key challenges in healthcare data management and proposes solutions to address them.

1. Data Security and Privacy: Challenge: Safeguarding patient data from unauthorized access, breaches, and cyber threats is a significant concern in healthcare data management. Stringent privacy regulations add an extra layer of complexity.

   Solution: Implement robust encryption, access controls, and authentication measures. Regular security audits and staff training on data security best practices are crucial. Adoption of advanced technologies like blockchain for secure, immutable record-keeping is also gaining traction.

2. Data Interoperability: Challenge: Healthcare data is often stored in disparate systems that do not seamlessly communicate with each other, leading to interoperability challenges. This hinders the efficient exchange of information among healthcare providers and systems.

   Solution: Promote the use of standardized data formats and interoperability standards (e.g., FHIR - Fast Healthcare

Interoperability Resources). Invest in health information exchange (HIE) platforms that facilitate secure sharing of patient data across different systems.

3. Data Quality and Accuracy: Challenge: Inaccurate or incomplete data can compromise patient care, research outcomes, and decision-making. Data quality issues may arise due to manual errors, inconsistent data entry, or outdated information.

   Solution: Implement data validation protocols, conduct regular audits, and employ automated tools for data cleansing. Encourage healthcare providers to adopt electronic health record (EHR) systems with built-in validation checks.

4. Scalability and Storage: Challenge: The growing volume of healthcare data, including electronic health records, medical imaging, and genomic data, poses challenges in terms of storage capacity and system scalability.

   Solution: Invest in scalable cloud-based storage solutions. Implement data archiving strategies to manage historical data efficiently. Regularly reassess storage needs and upgrade infrastructure accordingly.

5. Regulatory Compliance: Challenge: Healthcare data management must adhere to numerous regulatory standards, which vary globally. Keeping abreast of changing regulations and ensuring compliance is a constant challenge.

   Solution: Establish a dedicated compliance team, conduct regular training sessions, and implement compliance management tools. Leverage technology to automate compliance monitoring and reporting.

6. Data Governance and Ownership: Challenge: Determining clear ownership of healthcare data, defining access rights, and establishing governance structures are complex tasks. Lack of clear guidelines can lead to misuse or unauthorized access.

Solution: Develop robust data governance policies, clearly defining roles and responsibilities. Implement access controls and audit trails. Foster a culture of data stewardship, where all stakeholders understand their roles in ensuring data integrity.

7. Integration of Emerging Technologies: Challenge: Incorporating emerging technologies, such as artificial intelligence and blockchain, into healthcare data management requires overcoming technical and cultural barriers.

   Solution: Encourage collaboration between IT experts, healthcare professionals, and data scientists. Provide training programs to familiarize staff with new technologies. Start with pilot projects to assess feasibility and benefits.

8. Patient Consent and Engagement: Challenge: Obtaining and managing patient consent for data sharing and research participation can be challenging. Lack of patient engagement in managing their own health data is another hurdle.

   Solution: Implement transparent consent processes and utilize technology for secure patient engagement. Develop user-friendly interfaces for patients to access and manage their health information. Educate patients on the benefits of data sharing for improved healthcare outcomes.

9.8 Ethical Considerations and Patient Privacy

The evolving landscape of healthcare data management raises critical ethical considerations and underscores the importance of preserving patient privacy. The responsible handling of healthcare data is not only a legal requirement but also a moral obligation that directly impacts patient trust, autonomy, and the overall quality of healthcare services. Examining ethical considerations and patient privacy in the context of healthcare data management reveals the intricate balance required to harness the benefits of data-driven healthcare while safeguarding individual rights.

Informed Consent: Informed consent is the cornerstone of ethical healthcare data management. Patients have the right to be informed about how their data will be used, by whom, and for what purposes. This ensures that individuals are active participants in the decision-making process regarding their health information.

Implementation: Healthcare providers must establish transparent consent processes that educate patients about data collection, sharing, and potential uses. This involves clear communication, easy-to-understand language, and opportunities for patients to ask questions. Continuous efforts should be made to keep patients informed about any changes in data management practices.

Data Security and Confidentiality: Ensuring the security and confidentiality of healthcare data is an ethical imperative. Patients entrust their sensitive information to healthcare providers, expecting that it will be safeguarded against unauthorized access and breaches.

Implementation: Healthcare organizations must invest in robust cybersecurity measures, encryption protocols, and access controls to protect patient data. Regular training for healthcare staff on data security practices and the establishment of a culture of privacy contribute to maintaining confidentiality.

Data Sharing and Interoperability: The sharing of healthcare data with other entities or across systems raises ethical questions about consent, data accuracy, and the potential impact on patient privacy. Striking a balance between data sharing for improved patient care and respecting individual privacy rights is essential.

Implementation: Healthcare organizations should adopt interoperability standards and prioritize patient consent for data sharing. Clear policies and guidelines on data sharing practices, including de-identification methods, should be communicated to patients. Consent management tools can empower individuals to control the extent to which their data is shared.

Patient Access and Control: Respecting patients as owners of their health data requires providing them with access and control over their information. Empowering individuals to manage their data enhances autonomy and fosters a sense of ownership.

Implementation: Healthcare providers should offer secure patient portals, allowing individuals to access and review their health records. Tools for data correction and the ability to set preferences for data sharing contribute to patient control.

Long-Term Data Retention: Determining the appropriate duration for retaining healthcare data requires ethical considerations. Balancing the need for historical information with the right to privacy and the potential for data misuse is crucial.

Implementation: Healthcare organizations should establish and communicate clear data retention policies. Periodic reviews and purging of unnecessary data, especially outdated or irrelevant information, align with ethical principles and reduce the risk of unauthorized access.

Chapter
10

AI APPs IN HEALTHCARE

Various countries around the world have approved and implemented several AI applications in healthcare to improve patient care, enhance medical outcomes, and optimize healthcare delivery. Some of the notable AI applications in healthcare that have received regulatory approval or are in active use include

10.1 AI in Diagnostics

10.1.1 Medical Imaging Analysis

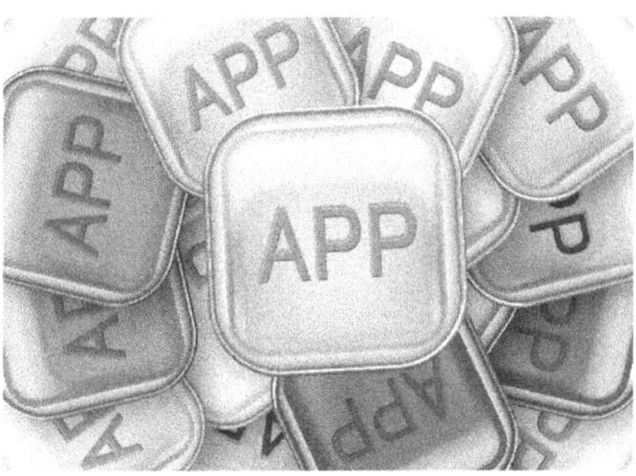

AI-powered algorithms for the analysis of medical imaging data, such as X-rays, CT scans, MRI scans, and mammograms, have been approved for clinical use in several countries. These applications assist radiologists in detecting abnormalities, diagnosing diseases, and providing more accurate interpretations of imaging studies. Recent innovations, like explainable AI, help build trust, while federated learning enables secure data exchange between institutions, fueling AI development. Together, AI and human expertise work in harmony to advance medical imaging, leading to improved patient care within healthcare analytics.

Example Product: FDA-cleared "IDx-DR" by IDx Technologies Inc. for autonomous detection of diabetic retinopathy using retinal images.

IDx-DR, or Intelligent Digital Radiography, represents a groundbreaking advancement in the field of medical imaging, specifically tailored to enhance the detection and diagnosis of diabetic retinopathy (DR). Diabetic retinopathy is a common complication of diabetes and a leading cause of blindness among working-age adults worldwide. IDx-DR utilizes artificial intelligence algorithms to analyse retinal images captured through digital imaging systems, offering a reliable and efficient method for early detection of diabetic retinopathy.

The technology behind IDx-DR is founded on deep learning algorithms, which are trained on vast datasets of retinal images to accurately identify signs of diabetic retinopathy. These algorithms are capable of detecting subtle abnormalities in retinal images indicative of diabetic retinopathy, such as microaneurysms, hemorrhages, and exudates, with high sensitivity and specificity.

One of the primary advantages of IDx-DR is its ability to provide autonomous image analysis, reducing the burden on healthcare professionals and facilitating widespread screening for diabetic retinopathy. The system operates autonomously, analysing retinal images without the need for direct human intervention. This autonomy not only improves efficiency but also enables healthcare providers to extend screening services to underserved populations or remote regions where access to specialized eye care may be limited.

Moreover, IDx-DR is designed to seamlessly integrate into existing clinical workflows, enhancing efficiency and scalability in diabetic retinopathy screening programs. Digital retinal images captured using standard fundus cameras are analysed in real-time by the IDx-DR software, which promptly provides diagnostic results indicating the presence or absence of diabetic retinopathy. This rapid turnaround time facilitates timely intervention and treatment, ultimately improving patient outcomes.

Another significant benefit of IDx-DR is its potential to reduce healthcare costs associated with diabetic retinopathy screening and management. By automating the screening process and minimizing the need for specialist intervention, IDx-DR offers a cost-effective solution for diabetic retinopathy screening on a large scale. Early detection and intervention facilitated by IDx-DR can also prevent the progression of diabetic retinopathy to advanced stages, reducing the economic burden of managing vision loss and blindness associated with the condition.

In addition to its clinical applications, IDx-DR exemplifies the transformative potential of AI in healthcare. The success of IDx-DR demonstrates the feasibility and efficacy of AI-driven diagnostic solutions in improving patient care and addressing unmet medical needs. Furthermore, IDx-DR serves as a model for the development and implementation of AI-based diagnostic tools across various medical specialties, paving the way for a future where AI augments healthcare delivery and enhances patient outcomes.

Following are some other top AI imaging tools

- Blackford: Delivers AI-enhanced medical image reconstruction that improves detail and reduces noise in CT scans.
- Viz.ai: Utilizes AI to assist in analysing chest X-rays, speeding up the detection of abnormalities and optimizing workflow.
- DeepMind AI for Radiography: Employs deep learning to automatically identify and segment anatomical structures in chest X-rays, aiding diagnosis and research.
- Arterys Medical: Provides cloud-based AI solutions for advanced visualization and analysis across various modalities, including CT, MRI, and ultrasound, with the goal of enhancing diagnostic accuracy and workflow.

10.1.2 Clinical Decision Support Systems (CDSS)

AI-driven clinical decision support systems offer real-time guidance to healthcare providers by analysing patient data and medical literature to assist in diagnosis, treatment planning, and medication selection. Some CDSS applications have received regulatory approval in countries like the United States, Europe, and Japan.

Example Product: "IBM Watson for Oncology" by IBM Corporation, providing evidence-based treatment recommendations for oncology patients

IBM Watson for Oncology is a pioneering cognitive computing platform designed to assist healthcare professionals in making evidence-based treatment decisions for cancer patients. Developed by IBM in collaboration with Memorial Sloan Kettering Cancer Center (MSK), Watson for Oncology leverages artificial intelligence and natural language processing (NLP) capabilities to analyse vast amounts of medical literature, clinical guidelines, patient records, and other relevant data sources to provide personalized treatment recommendations.

One of the primary objectives of Watson for Oncology is to address the complexity and variability inherent in cancer care by providing oncologists with access to the latest medical knowledge and evidence-based practices. The platform is trained on a comprehensive corpus of oncology literature, including medical journals, textbooks, treatment guidelines, and clinical trials data, enabling it to keep abreast of the latest advancements in cancer research and therapy.

Watson for Oncology operates by ingesting and analysing patient data, such as medical history, pathology reports, genomic profiles, and treatment options, and then generating personalized treatment recommendations based on the available evidence. The platform employs advanced algorithms to sift through vast amounts of information, identify relevant clinical insights, and present them in a format that is accessible and actionable for healthcare providers.

One of the key strengths of Watson for Oncology is its ability to provide tailored treatment recommendations that are aligned with established clinical guidelines and best practices. By integrating the latest evidence-based guidelines and expert knowledge from MSK, Watson for Oncology helps ensure that oncologists have access to the most up-to-date and relevant information when making treatment decisions for their patients.

Moreover, Watson for Oncology serves as a valuable decision support tool, empowering oncologists to make more informed and personalized treatment decisions. The platform presents oncologists with a comprehensive overview of treatment options, including potential benefits, risks, and considerations, allowing them to weigh the available evidence and tailor treatment plans to individual patient needs and preferences.

In addition to its clinical applications, Watson for Oncology also has the potential to improve healthcare efficiency and resource utilization. By automating aspects of the treatment decision-making process and providing oncologists with timely and relevant information, the platform can help streamline workflows, reduce decision-making time, and optimize resource allocation in oncology care settings.

However, it's essential to note that Watson for Oncology is not intended to replace the expertise of healthcare professionals but rather to augment their clinical judgment and decision-making process. While the platform can provide valuable insights and recommendations, the final treatment decisions remain the responsibility of the treating oncologist, who must consider the unique clinical context and preferences of each patient.

Following are some other top AI-driven clinical decision support systems

Oscar Health: Oscar Health utilizes AI and machine learning algorithms to personalize healthcare experiences, improve care coordination, and optimize health outcomes for its members. Its platform analyses patient data, clinical histories, and social determinants of health to deliver personalized care plans and preventive interventions.

Olive: Olive is an AI-driven healthcare automation platform that assists healthcare organizations in streamlining administrative tasks, revenue cycle management, and clinical workflows. It uses AI algorithms to automate repetitive tasks, optimize resource allocation, and enhance operational efficiency across the healthcare continuum.

VisualDx Clinical Pathways: VisualDx Clinical Pathways leverages AI algorithms to generate evidence-based clinical pathways and protocols for managing specific medical conditions and patient populations. It assists healthcare organizations in standardizing care practices, improving clinical outcomes, and reducing variations in treatment

10.2 AI in Monitoring

Remote Patient Monitoring: AI-enabled remote patient monitoring systems allow for continuous tracking of patients' vital signs, symptoms, and adherence to treatment plans outside of traditional healthcare settings. These systems help healthcare providers monitor patients remotely, detect early warning signs of deterioration, and intervene proactively to prevent adverse events. Some remote patient monitoring solutions have obtained regulatory approval in various countries.

Example Product: AI powered Apple Watch

The AI-powered Apple Watch represents a remarkable fusion of cutting-edge wearable technology and artificial intelligence, revolutionizing the way we monitor and manage our health and well-being. With each iteration, the Apple Watch has evolved to incorporate increasingly sophisticated AI capabilities, enhancing its ability to track and interpret user data for personalized insights and actionable recommendations.

At the heart of the AI-powered Apple Watch is its suite of advanced sensors and algorithms, which enable it to collect a wealth of health-related data in real-time. From heart rate and electrocardiogram (ECG)

measurements to activity levels and sleep patterns, the Apple Watch continuously monitors key physiological metrics, providing users with a comprehensive overview of their health and fitness.

One of the hallmark features of the AI-powered Apple Watch is its ability to analyse and interpret this data to deliver personalized health insights and recommendations. Using AI algorithms, the Apple Watch can detect irregularities in heart rhythm, identify trends in activity levels, and even predict potential health risks based on patterns in user data. These insights empower users to take proactive steps to improve their health and well-being, whether it's through adjusting their activity levels, seeking medical attention, or making lifestyle changes.

Furthermore, the AI-powered Apple Watch serves as a powerful tool for early detection and intervention in various health conditions. For example, the watch's ability to detect irregular heart rhythms, such as atrial fibrillation, can alert users to seek medical attention and potentially prevent serious cardiac events. Similarly, features like fall detection and emergency SOS can automatically summon help in the event of accidents or emergencies, providing users with added peace of mind.

In addition to its health monitoring capabilities, the AI-powered Apple Watch also offers a range of AI-driven features designed to enhance the user experience. From intelligent notifications and predictive text suggestions to personalized coaching and activity challenges, the watch leverages AI to adapt to users' preferences and behaviours, making it a truly personalized and intuitive companion for daily life.

Moreover, the AI-powered Apple Watch has the potential to revolutionize healthcare delivery by enabling remote patient monitoring and telemedicine services. By integrating with healthcare providers' systems and AI-driven analytics platforms, the watch can facilitate continuous monitoring of patients' health metrics, enabling early intervention and proactive management of chronic conditions.

Following are some other top AI-enabled remote patient monitoring systems:

WellDoc: This platform provides RPM for chronic conditions like diabetes and hypertension. It uses AI to analyse patient data (blood sugar readings, blood pressure readings) and offer personalized coaching and medication adjustments based on trends and risk factors

Tempus: This AI-powered platform focuses on remote patient monitoring after surgery. It analyses patient data (vitals, pain levels) and identifies potential complications, allowing for early intervention and improved recovery outcomes.

aliveCor: This company offers a smartphone-connected ECG device and an AI-powered app. The app analyses the user's ECG readings and can detect potential heart rhythm irregularities like atrial fibrillation.

AvaSure: AvaSure provides AI-enabled remote patient monitoring systems for healthcare facilities, particularly in intensive care units (ICUs) and behavioural health settings. Its platform utilizes video monitoring, motion detection, and machine learning algorithms to monitor patient movements, detect falls, and identify behavioural changes, enhancing patient safety and staff efficiency.

CarePredict: CarePredict offers an AI-driven remote monitoring solution for senior care facilities and home care settings. Its wearable sensor, called Tempo, continuously tracks activities of daily living (ADLs), sleep patterns, and social interactions to monitor seniors' health and well-being. Machine learning algorithms analyse the data to detect changes in behaviour and health status, providing early warning alerts to caregivers and family members.

10.3 AI in Treatment Planning

Personalized Medicine and Drug Discovery: AI algorithms are used to analyse genomic data, biomarkers, and other patient-specific information to tailor treatments and medications to individual patients. Additionally, AI is employed in drug discovery processes to identify potential drug candidates, predict drug responses, and accelerate the development of new therapies. Although specific AI-driven personalized medicine and drug discovery applications may not have regulatory approval, various AI-based technologies are actively used in these domains globally.

Example Product: One example of an AI application used for personalized medicine and drug discovery is "Atomwise

Atomwise is a company that utilizes AI-driven drug discovery technology to accelerate the process of identifying potential drug candidates for various diseases. Their platform employs deep learning algorithms to analyse molecular structures, predict interactions between compounds and biological targets, and prioritize promising drug candidates for further experimental validation.

Atomwise's AI technology enables virtual screening of millions of compounds against specific disease targets, allowing researchers to identify potential drug candidates with desirable properties, such as high potency, selectivity, and safety profiles. By leveraging AI for drug discovery, Atomwise aims to expedite the development of novel therapeutics and personalized treatment options for patients.

Following are some other similar AI applications:

Insilico Medicine: This AI platform utilizes deep learning for drug discovery and development. It can analyse vast datasets to identify potential drug candidates and predict their effectiveness for specific patients based on genetic and other factors.

Genoox: Genoox provides a cloud-based genomic analysis platform that incorporates AI algorithms to interpret genetic data and generate actionable insights for personalized medicine. Its platform uses machine learning techniques to identify clinically relevant variants, assess disease risks, and recommend targeted therapies based on individuals' genetic profiles

Deep Genomics: Deep Genomics utilizes AI algorithms to analyse genetic data and predict how genetic variations impact disease risk, treatment response, and drug efficacy. Its platform combines genomics data with biological knowledge and machine learning models to identify disease-causing mutations and develop personalized treatment strategies.

Natural Language Processing (NLP): NLP algorithms extract and analyse information from unstructured clinical notes, electronic health records (EHRs), and medical literature to support various healthcare tasks, such as clinical documentation, coding, and research. While NLP applications themselves may not require regulatory approval, they are integral components of AI-driven healthcare solutions approved for clinical use in multiple countries.

Example Product: "Cerner Natural Language Processing" by Cerner Corporation, an NLP tool for extracting clinical insights from unstructured EHR data.

Cerner Natural Language Processing (NLP) is an advanced technology developed by Cerner Corporation, a leading provider of healthcare information technology solutions. This NLP solution is designed to extract valuable insights from unstructured clinical text data within electronic health records (EHRs) and other healthcare documents. By harnessing the power of natural language processing algorithms, Cerner NLP enables healthcare organizations to unlock the wealth of information embedded in narrative clinical notes, reports, and documentation.

At its core, Cerner NLP employs sophisticated machine learning and linguistic analysis techniques to parse, understand, and interpret free-text clinical data. This includes physician notes, radiology reports, pathology reports, discharge summaries, and other forms of unstructured clinical documentation. By automatically extracting relevant clinical concepts, entities, and relationships from these textual sources, Cerner NLP helps healthcare providers uncover actionable insights that can inform clinical decision-making, support quality improvement initiatives, and drive research efforts.

The key features and capabilities of Cerner NLP include:

1. Clinical Data Abstraction: Cerner NLP automatically identifies and extracts pertinent clinical information from unstructured text, such as patient demographics, medical history, diagnoses, procedures, medications, laboratory results, and clinical assessments.
2. Semantic Understanding: The NLP algorithms employed by Cerner can comprehend the context, semantics, and nuances of clinical language, enabling accurate extraction of clinical concepts and relationships from diverse healthcare documents.
3. Coding Assistance: Cerner NLP aids in clinical coding and documentation by suggesting appropriate diagnostic codes, procedure codes, and billing codes based on the extracted clinical information, streamlining the coding process and ensuring accurate reimbursement.
4. Clinical Decision Support: By analysing clinical narratives and identifying relevant clinical findings, Cerner NLP supports clinical decision-making by providing contextually relevant information to healthcare providers at the point of care. This may include alerting clinicians to potential drug-drug interactions, adverse events, or missing clinical data.
5. Quality Reporting and Research: Cerner NLP facilitates quality reporting initiatives and clinical research endeavors by enabling comprehensive analysis of large volumes of unstructured clinical data. It empowers healthcare organizations to derive meaningful insights from textual documentation, identify trends, assess outcomes, and conduct retrospective studies to inform evidence-based practice.

Following are some other similar NLP Applications

Ada Health: Uses NLP to provide patients with personalized health assessments and symptom checking.

cTAKES (clinical Text Analysis and Knowledge Extraction System): An open-source NLP system for information extraction from electronic medical records.

MedLEE (Medical Language Extraction and Encoding): A tool for extracting structured information from narrative medical reports.

10.4 Robot-Assisted Surgery

AI-powered robotic surgical systems assist surgeons in performing minimally invasive procedures with enhanced precision, dexterity, and control. Several robotic surgical systems have received regulatory clearance or approval for specific surgical procedures in various countries.

Example Product: "da Vinci Surgical System" by Intuitive Surgical Inc., a robotic surgical platform for minimally invasive procedures across various surgical specialties.

The da Vinci Surgical System is often described as a robotic surgical system rather than an artificial intelligence application. While it incorporates advanced technologies and automation, including robotic arms and sophisticated imaging, it does not typically utilize AI in the same way that some other systems might.

The system's functionality primarily relies on the surgeon's direct control and manipulation of the robotic arms from a console. The surgeon's movements are translated into precise actions by the robotic arms, allowing for enhanced dexterity and precision during surgery. However, these actions are guided entirely by the surgeon's inputs and commands rather than autonomous decision-making by AI algorithms.

That said, Intuitive Surgical, the company behind the da Vinci system, continually works on enhancing its technologies, and there may be elements of AI integrated into newer iterations or future developments of the system. For example, AI could potentially be used for tasks such as image analysis, surgical planning, or decision support. However, as of my last update, the da Vinci Surgical System is primarily recognized for its robotic and imaging technologies rather than AI-based functionalities.

Following are some other similar Applications:

MAKOplasty: The MAKO system is designed for orthopedic surgery, particularly for partial knee resurfacing and total hip and knee replacements. It uses a combination of 3D imaging and robotic arm technology.

CyberKnife: The CyberKnife system is a robotic radiosurgery system used for non-invasive treatment of tumors. It delivers high doses of radiation with sub-millimeter accuracy.

ExcelsiusGPS®: ExcelsiusGPS is a robotic navigation platform designed to improve the safety and accuracy of spinal surgery. It integrates navigation and robotic guidance for precise placement of implants.

Healthcare Chatbots and Virtual Assistants: AI-driven chatbots and virtual assistants provide patients with personalized health advice, symptom triage, appointment scheduling, medication reminders, and telemedicine consultations. Some healthcare chatbot platforms have obtained regulatory clearance or approval for use in specific healthcare contexts.

Example Product: “Buoy Health” by Buoy Health Inc., an AI-powered chatbot for symptom checking, triage, and personalized health recommendations.

Buoy Health is an innovative healthcare technology company that leverages artificial intelligence to provide personalized health information and guidance to users. Founded in 2014 by a team of doctors, data scientists, and engineers, Buoy Health aims to improve access to healthcare resources and empower individuals to make informed decisions about their health.

The Buoy Health platform operates primarily through a user-friendly chat interface, where individuals can input their symptoms and receive personalized recommendations and information. Here's an overview of Buoy Health's features and functionalities:

1. Symptom Assessment: Users can describe their symptoms to Buoy Health through the chat interface. The platform utilizes AI algorithms, natural language processing (NLP), and a vast database of medical knowledge to assess the severity and potential causes of the reported symptoms.
2. Personalized Recommendations: Based on the information provided by the user, Buoy Health generates personalized recommendations and next steps. This may include advice on self-care measures, suggestions for when to seek medical attention, and information about possible conditions associated with the reported symptoms.
3. Referral to Care: If necessary, Buoy Health can help users find nearby healthcare providers or schedule appointments with doctors. It provides information about local healthcare services and facilities, including urgent care centers and hospitals.
4. Continuous Learning: Buoy Health's AI continuously learns from user interactions and feedback to improve its accuracy and effectiveness over time. It adapts its responses based on new information and updates in medical knowledge, ensuring that users receive the most relevant and up-to-date guidance.
5. Focus on Accessibility and Equity: Buoy Health is committed to improving healthcare access and reducing disparities by providing free, accessible, and inclusive services. The platform is available online and through mobile devices, allowing users to access healthcare information anytime, anywhere.

Following are some other similar Applications:

WebMD Symptom Checker: WebMD offers an online symptom checker tool that helps users understand possible causes of their symptoms and provides information on treatments and next steps.

Symptoma: Symptoma provides an AI-powered symptom checker that helps users identify potential conditions based on their symptoms. It generates a report that users can share with healthcare providers.

Your.MD: A health information platform with an AI-based symptom checker providing condition insights and self-care advice.

Chapter 11

AI START-UPS IN HEALTHCARE

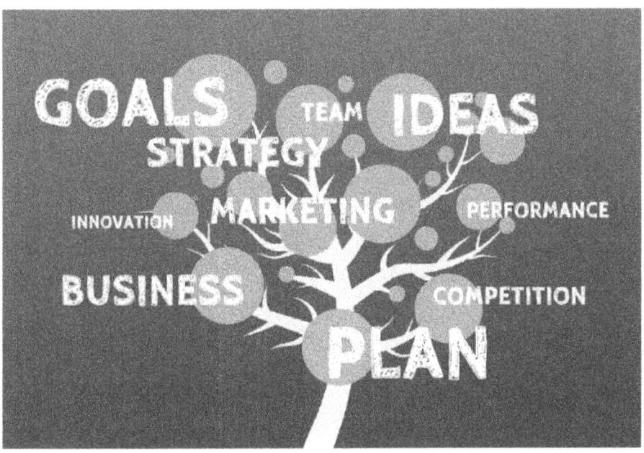

A startup is typically defined as a newly established business enterprise in its early stages of development. Startups are characterized by their innovative business model, product, or service offerings, often leveraging new technology or a novel approach to solving a problem. The AI startup ecosystem thrives on innovation, but it's also fraught with obstacles that test the resilience and adaptability of emerging companies. The challenges encompass both technical aspects, such as creating reliable algorithms and handling large datasets, and business-related issues, including clearly communicating value propositions and engaging stakeholders. For AI startups, moving from an idea to a marketable product is herculean task. It demands patience, persistence, and a deep understanding of the technology and market environment. Key characteristics of startups include:

- Innovation: Startups introduce new products, services, or business models that differentiate them from existing offerings in the market.
- High Growth Potential: Startups aim for rapid growth and scalability, seeking to expand their customer base and market reach quickly.

- Risk and Uncertainty: Startups operate in an environment of uncertainty, facing risks related to market acceptance, funding, competition, and operational challenges.
- Entrepreneurial Spirit: Startups are typically founded by entrepreneurs or small teams with a vision to disrupt industries or create significant impact.
- Limited Resources: Startups often operate with limited financial resources and manpower initially, requiring them to be resourceful and agile in their operations.
- Focus on Problem Solving: Startups are driven by solving specific problems or addressing unmet needs in the market, often targeting niche or underserved segments.

A profound yet quiet revolution is underway in healthcare, fuelled by the innovative power of Artificial Intelligence. At the forefront of this change are AI healthcare startups, spearheading this new era of medical advancements. These startups aren't just part of the healthcare landscape; they're actively reshaping it, offering solutions that once belonged to the realm of science fiction. More than just technology firms, these ventures are visionaries, using AI to address intricate problems, create new markets, and provide unparalleled solutions.

11.1 Opportunities Offered by AI Healthcare Start-ups

Healthcare startups are revolutionizing the medical sector through the integration of AI, presenting solutions that are set to transform patient care, improve operational efficiencies, and increase global accessibility to healthcare. Here's a look at the advancements these AI-driven startups are bringing to the medical field.

1. Improve Patient Outcomes: AI-driven healthcare startups are at the forefront of precision medicine, utilizing advanced data analysis to sift through extensive medical data for more accurate

diagnoses and personalized treatment plans. This approach significantly enhances patient outcomes by offering healthcare solutions that are both highly efficient and tailored to the unique needs of each patient, representing a notable advancement in the delivery of medical care.

2. Operational Efficiency: AI healthcare startups are enhancing the efficiency of healthcare facilities by automating administrative tasks such as scheduling, billing, and managing patient records. By handling these time-consuming responsibilities, AI systems free up healthcare providers to concentrate on delivering patient care. This transition not only boosts the quality of care but also heightens satisfaction among patients and providers by reducing administrative burdens and making services more responsive.
3. Cost Reduction: AI healthcare startups have been leading the charge in reducing healthcare costs by streamlining operational processes and cutting down on unnecessary tests and procedures. This approach not only alleviates financial pressures on healthcare systems, making healthcare more accessible to patients, but also supports the sustainability of healthcare providers, ensuring that quality services remain available when needed.
4. Innovative Treatment Solutions: The integration of AI in healthcare has paved the way for groundbreaking treatment options, with AI healthcare startups spearheading advancements in drug discovery and the customization of therapy plans for individual patients. This progress not only enhances the quality of care but also accelerates the time it takes to bring new treatments to market, leading to improved patient outcomes and overall success.
5. Global Healthcare Access: AI healthcare startups are crucial in expanding healthcare access to underserved and remote regions through the use of AI-powered diagnostic tools and telemedicine services. These technologies overcome geographical and logistical obstacles, making high-quality healthcare services more accessible

to global populations. This enhanced access is essential for bridging health disparity gaps and ensuring that everyone has the opportunity to receive quality medical care, no matter where they are located and what their financial status is.

11.2 Challenges of Implementing AI into Healthcare Settings

1. Deficiency of Internal Expertise: A shortage of in-house expertise can significantly impede a startup's ability to innovate and develop effective AI-driven solutions. For instance, a startup aiming to transform healthcare with AI might face challenges without the necessary combination of AI researchers and healthcare specialists. To overcome this, startups are increasingly engaging in strategic hiring, forming partnerships with academic institutions, and investing in training programs for their current teams. An AI Design Agency can expedite your startup's progress by applying expert design strategies. Harvard Business Review highlights case studies where top AI startups have advanced their innovation through strategic partnerships. This method not only boosts their capabilities but also promotes a culture of ongoing learning and innovation.
2. Infrastructure Constraints: AI technologies require significant computing power and data storage capabilities, which can pose a major barrier to entry. High-performance GPUs and extensive data storage are essential but costly. Many startups are addressing this challenge by utilizing cloud computing services, which provide scalable and flexible resources at a lower cost than investing in physical hardware. This approach allows startups to concentrate on developing and scaling their solutions without the burden of substantial upfront expenses.

   Training, testing, and deploying AI systems can be costly, with expenses related to dataset collection, computing power, and storage. Many healthcare organizations also lack the necessary data infrastructure to gather and utilize data effectively for training algorithms, testing for biases, and ongoing model adjustments. The absence of digital infrastructure further complicates the development of AI systems.

3. Access to data: AI systems rely on access to extensive datasets, which presents a significant challenge for developing indigenous AI solutions in many developing countries and even in some developed nations. Healthcare data is usually fragmented, scattered, and often incomplete. Effective AI development requires longitudinal data, but patients frequently visit different doctors for the same condition or treatment, leading to a lack of continuity. Many healthcare providers are informal and unaccredited, resulting in non-standardized data collection and varying approaches to medical care.

   Insufficient digitization in hospitals complicates the situation further. It is common for patients to be assigned new registration numbers or files with each visit, and prescriptions are often handwritten. Frontline health workers typically record patient histories in notebooks using their own methods. Consequently, the data available for AI companies is likely to be unrepresentative of a significant portion of the population.
4. Data Collection Gaps: Current AI experiments rely heavily on historical data from specific hospitals or research institutions. The issue with historical data, as highlighted in existing AI studies, is that it inherently reflects societal biases and discrimination (Gershgorn, 2018). For instance, there are documented cases where women from lower castes have been denied healthcare due to class elitism among medical providers (Siddiqui, 2008). Additionally, clinical trial data used for AI development often under-represents women, minorities, and the elderly, as these groups are less frequently included in trials (Hart, 2017). Consequently, medicines developed from such data may be

effective only for certain populations. Algorithms trained on these datasets may thus have significant blind spots, potentially leading to misdiagnosis in extreme cases.

5. Data Privacy and Security: One of the major challenges is protecting patient data. AI systems access vast quantities of sensitive health information, which raises concerns about potential breaches or misuse. Hospitals and medical organizations need to invest in strong cybersecurity measures to safeguard patient information and comply with government regulations. Best practices involve using advanced encryption techniques and following privacy regulations closely.
6. Interoperability and Data Standardization: The lack of standardization in healthcare data formats and interoperability issues between different systems can create significant challenges for AI applications and products. For AI to function effectively, it needs access to comprehensive, standardized data across various healthcare platforms.
7. Ethical and Legal Considerations: The use of AI in healthcare brings up ethical concerns regarding decision-making and accountability, especially when it comes to diagnosis or treatment decisions. To gain widespread acceptance, AI systems must address both legal and ethical issues.
8. Skill Gap and Training: Given the growing skills gap in healthcare professions regarding AI technology, it is essential to train healthcare workers in utilizing and interpreting AI-generated insights to fully benefit from these advancements.

By tackling these challenges directly, AI startups can establish a strong foundation for growth and success. The crucial factor is to identify these obstacles early and adopt strategic approaches to address them, whether by utilizing external resources, building partnerships, or prioritizing data security and privacy from the outset.

11.3 Strategic Imperatives for AI Start-ups in Healthcare

1. Appreciate business model very early: For AI startups in healthcare, grasping the business model from the outset is essential for long-term success. Early comprehension of the business model enables startups to align their AI solutions with market needs, regulatory requirements, and revenue generation strategies. This understanding helps in defining the target audience, identifying key value propositions, and setting realistic goals for product development and commercialization. By focusing on the business model early, AI startups can optimize their approach, attract investors, and build partnerships that are aligned with their strategic vision. This proactive approach lays a solid foundation for growth and helps navigate the complexities of the healthcare landscape more effectively.
2. Spotting Opportunities for AI Integration: Identifying key areas where AI can make a difference is essential. Successful examples often come from startups that thoughtfully incorporate AI to improve their main services or products. For instance, a startup specializing in customer service might use natural language processing (NLP) to automate responses to frequently asked questions, greatly decreasing response times and boosting customer satisfaction. Another example involves using AI for predictive analytics in supply chain management, which helps optimize inventory levels based on predictive models. These examples underscore the value of strategically integrating AI in ways that align with business objectives and produce clear benefits.
3. Standing Out in a Competitive Field: Startups can set themselves apart by focusing on niche markets, creating unique technology, or providing exceptional customer experiences. By addressing specific industry problems or offering highly personalized user interactions, a startup can distinguish itself from the competition.

Effective differentiation relies on a deep understanding of customer needs and clearly demonstrating how your AI solutions provide unique benefits compared to rivals.

4. Collaborations Are Essential: Successful partnerships can provide access to essential resources and expertise, simplifying the journey to innovation and market entry. They allow startups to utilize established infrastructures, data sources, and funding opportunities, easing the initial challenges of resource acquisition.
5. Work with healthcare professionals: Expanding on the significance of working with healthcare professionals, their expertise is vital in creating a healthcare product or service. From the early stages of brainstorming to the final launch, these professionals can offer critical insights into industry challenges, share valuable experiences, and highlight areas needing enhancement. They also assist entrepreneurs in grasping the regulatory framework, navigating the intricate healthcare environment, and accessing essential resources and networks.
6. Show Scalability and Market Fit: To attract investors, it's crucial to achieve a clear product-market fit and show that your business can scale. This requires thorough market research, gathering customer feedback, and adjusting your product to effectively address the identified needs.
7. Shift from Point to Platform: Hospitals prefer integrated platform solutions over narrow point solutions. While current AI applications often address specific diseases or workflow steps, hospitals seek comprehensive platforms that seamlessly connect systems and departments, facilitating coordinated patient care and reducing the complexity of managing multiple point solutions.
8. Protect Your Innovations: Patents, trademarks, and copyrights protect your innovations, minimize competition, and boost your valuation with investors and partners. For AI in healthcare startups, intellectual property (IP) is crucial, especially when

creating proprietary algorithms or using external data. Effectively managing and understanding IP rights is vital for establishing your startup's value and building trust with partners and customers.

9. Target Niche Markets: Focusing on niche markets in healthcare startups allows for the development of specialized solutions that directly address unique needs, leading to improved patient outcomes and satisfaction. This targeted approach reduces competition by concentrating on less saturated segments, enabling startups to establish themselves as leaders in their specific field. Additionally, it streamlines resource allocation and operational efficiency by allowing startups to focus their efforts and expertise on a defined area, ultimately accelerating time-to-market and enhancing overall business performance.
10. Validate Early: The key to successful innovation is early validation of your AI solution with both end-users and hospital decision-makers. Innovators often focus heavily on developing their technology, but it's crucial to balance this with a deep understanding of the actual problem and a broader perspective on its scope.
11. Staying Updated on AI Innovations: The AI sector is advancing rapidly, so it's essential for startups to keep up with the latest technologies and methods. Staying updated involves continuous learning, participating in industry conferences, and interacting with the AI research community. To stay ahead, startups must be proactive in their innovation efforts, committed to continuous learning, and adaptable to emerging trends and technologies
12. Navigate Regulatory Compliance: Healthcare is one of the most heavily regulated sectors worldwide, so entrepreneurs need a thorough understanding of regulatory requirements. They must be ready to dedicate time and resources to ensure their products or services comply with these standards. Non-compliance can lead to substantial fines, penalties, and legal challenges. Hence, collaborating closely with legal and regulatory experts is crucial

to ensure that your product or service adheres to all required regulations

13. Resource Allocation: Balancing the budget with AI development needs is a key challenge for startups. AI projects demand substantial investments in talent, technology, and data. Startups must prioritize high-ROI projects, seek external funding or partnerships, and use lean development methods to optimize resource allocation. This approach helps sustain AI development while scaling operations efficiently.
14. Funding: Securing funding for pre-revenue healthcare startups is particularly challenging due to high development, regulatory and clinical trial costs. Entrepreneurs need to present a strong business case and a clear path to profitability to attract investors. It's crucial to target investors who understand the healthcare industry, as they will be more familiar with the necessary funding requirements and can provide valuable industry connections. This focus can streamline the funding process and avoid unnecessary discussions

11.4 Glimpses on Startups

Here are some notable startups across countries harnessing AI to drive transformative changes in healthcare. These innovative companies are pushing the boundaries of technology to enhance diagnostic accuracy, personalize treatments, and improve overall patient outcomes.

1. Niramai: Niramai is a pioneering health tech startup focused on revolutionizing breast cancer screening through AI-driven technology. Their innovative solution uses machine learning and thermal imaging to provide a non-invasive, radiation-free method for early detection, aiming to make breast cancer screening more accessible and effective, particularly in underserved regions.
2. HealthifyMe: This is a dynamic health and wellness startup that leverages AI to offer personalized fitness and nutrition guidance. By combining advanced algorithms with real-time data, the

platform delivers tailored recommendations, tracks progress, and provides virtual coaching, helping users achieve their health goals more effectively and sustainably.

3. Olive AI: Olive AI is a forward-thinking startup that focuses on automating administrative and operational tasks within healthcare systems using artificial intelligence. By streamlining processes such as billing, patient scheduling, and data management, Olive AI aims to reduce operational inefficiencies and allow healthcare professionals to concentrate more on patient care.
4. Babylon Health: Babylon Health is an innovative digital health startup that integrates AI to deliver comprehensive and accessible healthcare solutions. Through its platform, Babylon offers virtual consultations, symptom checkers, and personalized health insights, aiming to make high-quality medical care more convenient and available to a global audience.
5. Qure.ai: A cutting-edge startup specializing in AI-powered diagnostic solutions for medical imaging. Their technology uses advanced algorithms to analyse radiological images, providing accurate and rapid insights for conditions like tuberculosis and brain disorders, thereby enhancing diagnostic efficiency and supporting healthcare providers in delivering timely and precise care
6. Atomwise: This is an innovative startup that leverages artificial intelligence to advance drug discovery. By employing deep learning algorithms to analyse molecular interactions, Atomwise accelerates the identification of promising drug candidates and optimizes their potential efficacy. This approach aims to streamline the drug development process and uncover new treatments more efficiently.
7. Wysa: Wysa is a pioneering mental health startup that leverages AI to offer accessible and personalized emotional support. Through its chatbot-based platform, Wysa provides users with evidence-based therapeutic techniques, mental wellness exercises, and real-

time emotional support, aiming to enhance mental well-being and provide scalable mental health solutions.

8. Beijing Infervision: Beijing Infervision empowers radiologists, surgeons, researchers and healthcare teams with intuitive, comprehensive AI solutions that improve patient outcomes and streamline hospital operations. Provide advanced AI solutions that assist medical professionals across all facets of healthcare, including disease screening and diagnosis, treatment and intervention, patient management, and medical research.
9. Symptoma: Symptoma is an innovative health tech startup that utilizes AI to assist users in identifying potential medical conditions based on their symptoms. By analysing user-reported symptoms and medical data, Symptoma provides a differential diagnosis and helps guide individuals towards appropriate medical consultations, aiming to enhance early detection and improve overall healthcare efficiency.
10. Biofourmis: Biofourmis integrates wearable sensors, advanced analytics, and machine learning to monitor patient health and manage chronic conditions. Their flagship platform, Biovitals™, combines data from these wearable devices with sophisticated algorithms to provide real-time health monitoring and predictive analytics. This approach allows healthcare providers to make more informed decisions, improve patient outcomes, and enhance the overall efficiency of care delivery.

Chapter 12

AI IN HEALTHCARE-MYTH AND REALITY

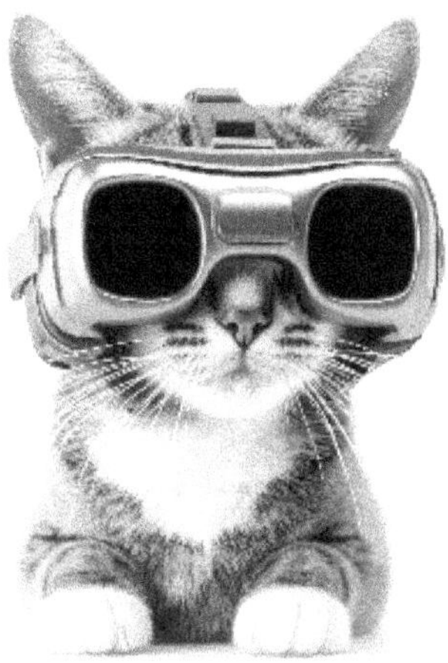

In preceding chapters, we have explored the burgeoning influence of Artificial Intelligence in healthcare, unveiling its transformative potential across diagnostics, treatment modalities, and patient care. From precision medicine to predictive analytics, AI offers a plethora of opportunities to revolutionize the healthcare landscape. However, amid the hype, it's crucial to discern between the myths surrounding AI in healthcare and the practical realities of its implementation. This chapter embarks on a comprehensive exploration of AI's role in healthcare, delving into prevalent myths, dissecting implementation challenges, and unraveling the nuanced realities shaping its integration into the industry.

12.1 Myths Surrounding AI in Healthcare

12.1.1. AI Will Replace Doctors

The widespread myth that AI will render human physicians obsolete is a fallacy rooted in misconceptions about AI's capabilities. While AI augments diagnostic accuracy and aids in treatment decisions, it cannot replicate the holistic approach and empathetic care provided by healthcare professionals. Rather than displacing doctors, AI serves as a supportive tool, enhancing their expertise and improving patient outcomes through data-driven insights.

AI excels in tasks that involve pattern recognition, data analysis, and repetitive processes. For example, AI algorithms can swiftly analyse vast amounts of medical imaging data, identifying potential abnormalities more quickly and accurately than human eyes alone. In addition, AI systems can integrate and process diverse datasets from electronic health records, genomic information, and clinical research to support evidence-based decision-making.

However, the practice of medicine involves much more than data analysis. Physicians provide personalized care that considers the patient's unique circumstances, emotional state, and social context. They engage in nuanced clinical reasoning, communicate complex information compassionately, and make ethical decisions in situations where guidelines may not provide clear answers. These aspects of patient care require empathy, judgment, and human interaction—qualities that AI cannot replicate.

Moreover, AI in healthcare is designed to function as an assistive technology. By automating routine tasks and providing decision support, AI can free up healthcare professionals to focus more on direct patient care and complex decision-making. For instance, AI can handle administrative tasks like scheduling, documentation, and billing, reducing the clerical burden on physicians and allowing them to spend more time with patients.

Additionally, AI tools can act as second opinions, providing doctors with additional perspectives on diagnostic and treatment options. This collaborative approach leverages the strengths of both AI and human expertise, leading to more accurate diagnoses, personalized treatment plans, and ultimately better patient outcomes.

The integration of AI into healthcare also emphasizes the importance of multidisciplinary teams. AI developers, data scientists, and healthcare professionals work together to design and implement AI systems that align with clinical needs and ethical standards. This collaboration ensures that AI tools are not only technically robust but also clinically relevant and user-friendly.

Furthermore, the education and training of healthcare professionals increasingly include aspects of AI and data science. This empowers doctors to understand and leverage AI tools effectively, ensuring they remain at the forefront of medical innovation while maintaining the central role of human judgment and patient interaction in healthcare.

In summary, the notion that AI will replace doctors is a myth. AI enhances the capabilities of healthcare professionals by providing powerful tools for data analysis and decision support, allowing them to deliver more effective and compassionate care. Far from being a threat, AI represents an opportunity to elevate the practice of medicine, benefiting both doctors and patients alike.

12.1.2. AI is Infallible

The portrayal of AI as an infallible diagnostician overlooks its inherent limitations and vulnerabilities. While AI systems can significantly enhance diagnostic accuracy and provide valuable insights, they are far from perfect and must be approached with a critical eye. Several factors contribute to the fallibility of AI in healthcare:

1. Biases in Training Data: AI models are trained on historical data, and if this data is biased or unrepresentative, the AI will inherit and potentially amplify these biases. For example, if a dataset predominantly features data from a specific demographic group, the AI might perform poorly on underrepresented populations, leading to disparities in healthcare outcomes. Biases in data can result from various sources, including socio-economic factors, racial disparities, and sampling errors.

2. Algorithmic Errors: Algorithms can make mistakes, especially when faced with ambiguous or borderline cases. Misclassification, overfitting, and underfitting are common issues in machine learning that can lead to incorrect predictions. For instance, an AI system might misinterpret a benign anomaly as malignant in a medical image, resulting in unnecessary anxiety and further testing for the patient.
3. Lack of Contextual Understanding: AI lacks the ability to understand context in the way humans do. While it can analyse patterns in data, it doesn't grasp the nuances of patient history, lifestyle, and other contextual factors that are crucial for accurate diagnosis and treatment planning. For example, a patient's symptoms might be influenced by psychological or social factors that an AI system, focused purely on physiological data, might miss.
4. Intuitive Reasoning and Clinical Judgment: Experienced healthcare professionals possess intuitive reasoning and clinical judgment honed through years of practice. These skills enable them to make decisions in complex, uncertain situations where guidelines may not provide clear answers. AI lacks this human intuition and the ability to weigh various factors in real-time decision-making. For instance, a doctor might choose a less aggressive treatment approach based on their knowledge of a patient's overall health and preferences, a nuance that an AI might overlook.
5. Vulnerability to Adversarial Attacks: AI systems can be susceptible to adversarial attacks, where deliberately altered inputs cause the AI to make incorrect predictions. In healthcare, such vulnerabilities could be exploited to manipulate diagnostic outcomes or treatment recommendations, posing serious risks to patient safety.
6. Dynamic and Evolving Nature of Medicine: Medicine is constantly evolving with new research, treatments, and guidelines emerging regularly. AI systems need continuous updates and retraining to

stay current with the latest medical knowledge. Without regular updates, an AI system's recommendations might become outdated, leading to suboptimal or even harmful advice.

7. Ethical and Regulatory Challenges: Implementing AI in healthcare involves navigating complex ethical and regulatory landscapes. Ensuring patient privacy, data security, and obtaining regulatory approval for AI tools are significant challenges that can impact the reliability and acceptance of AI solutions.

In summary, while AI holds great promise for transforming healthcare, it is not infallible. Recognizing its limitations and ensuring robust human oversight is essential for the safe and effective integration of AI into clinical practice.

12.1.3. AI Will Reduce Healthcare Costs Overnight

Expectations of immediate cost savings through AI implementation oversimplify the intricate dynamics of healthcare economics. While AI holds the potential to streamline processes, reduce errors, and optimize resource utilization, its integration requires substantial investments in infrastructure, training, and regulatory compliance. Furthermore, the long-term impact on healthcare costs hinges on various factors, including adoption rates, reimbursement models, and healthcare policy reforms. Here are several key reasons why the expectation of instant cost reductions is unrealistic:

1. Initial Investment Costs: Implementing AI in healthcare necessitates substantial initial investments. This includes purchasing advanced software and hardware, upgrading existing IT infrastructure, and integrating AI systems with current electronic health records (EHR) and other clinical tools. Additionally, there are costs associated with data storage and processing, especially for large-scale applications like medical imaging and genomic analysis.
2. Training and Workforce Development: Successful AI deployment requires training healthcare professionals to

effectively use AI tools. This involves educating doctors, nurses, and administrative staff on how to interpret AI-generated insights and integrate them into clinical workflows. Furthermore, ongoing professional development is necessary to keep pace with advancements in AI technology and ensure that staff can utilize these tools effectively.

3. Regulatory Compliance and Validation: AI systems in healthcare must comply with stringent regulatory standards to ensure patient safety and data privacy. Meeting these regulatory requirements involves thorough validation and certification processes, which can be time-consuming and costly. Additionally, maintaining compliance with evolving regulations requires continuous monitoring and adjustments to the AI systems.
4. Integration Challenges: Integrating AI into existing healthcare systems is a complex task that involves significant technical and organizational challenges. Ensuring interoperability between AI tools and various healthcare databases and systems is crucial for seamless functionality. This integration process can be lengthy and resource-intensive, potentially delaying the realization of cost savings.
5. Long-Term Savings Potential: While AI can potentially reduce healthcare costs in the long term by improving efficiency, reducing medical errors, and optimizing resource utilization, these benefits may not be immediately apparent. For instance, AI can help reduce hospital readmissions and streamline administrative processes, but the financial impact of these improvements will accumulate over time.
6. Variable Adoption Rates: The pace at which AI is adopted across different healthcare settings varies significantly. Factors influencing adoption rates include organizational readiness, availability of resources, and the perceived value of AI tools by healthcare providers. Early adopters may experience initial setbacks and learning curves that can affect cost savings.

7. Reimbursement Models: The impact of AI on healthcare costs is also influenced by existing reimbursement models. For example, fee-for-service models might not incentivize the use of AI tools aimed at preventative care and efficiency. On the other hand, value-based care models, which reward healthcare providers for quality and outcomes, might be more conducive to realizing cost savings through AI.
8. Healthcare Policy Reforms: The broader economic impact of AI in healthcare is contingent on supportive healthcare policies and reforms. Policies that promote innovation, provide funding for AI research, and incentivize the adoption of AI technologies can accelerate cost-saving benefits. Conversely, regulatory barriers and lack of policy support can hinder progress.
9. Maintenance and Upgrades: AI systems require regular maintenance, updates, and upgrades to remain effective and secure. These ongoing costs need to be factored into the overall economic evaluation of AI in healthcare. Neglecting maintenance can lead to system failures, data breaches, and reduced effectiveness, potentially increasing costs instead of reducing them.

In summary, while AI holds significant promise for reducing healthcare costs by enhancing efficiency, minimizing errors, and optimizing resource use, the expectation of immediate cost savings is unrealistic. The journey to realizing the full economic benefits of AI in healthcare involves substantial upfront investments, comprehensive training, and a supportive regulatory and policy environment. The long-term impact on healthcare costs will depend on various factors, including how quickly and effectively AI is adopted, integrated, and supported by healthcare systems and policies.

12.1.4. AI Will Solve All Medical Mysteries

The portrayal of AI as a panacea for medical discovery underestimates the complexities of scientific research and clinical practice. While AI accelerates data analysis and pattern recognition, it cannot replace the creativity, curiosity, and expertise of human researchers and clinicians. Medical breakthroughs require interdisciplinary collabouration, rigorous experimentation, and serendipitous insights, with AI serving as a facilitator rather than a substitute for human ingenuity. Here are several key reasons why AI alone cannot solve all medical mysteries:

1. Complexity of Medical Research: Medical research is inherently complex, involving not just data analysis but also hypothesis generation, experimental design, and clinical trials. While AI can process vast amounts of data to identify patterns and generate hypotheses, it lacks the capacity for the intuitive leaps and creative thinking that often drive groundbreaking discoveries. Human researchers are essential for designing experiments, interpreting results in context, and making novel connections that AI might miss.
2. Interdisciplinary Collaboration: Medical breakthroughs typically result from the collaboration of diverse teams, including clinicians, researchers, engineers, and patients. AI can facilitate this collaboration by providing tools for data sharing and analysis, but it cannot replace the human element of teamwork and communication. Successful medical discoveries often emerge from the synergy of different perspectives and expertise, something that AI alone cannot achieve.
3. Rigorous Experimentation: Scientific advancements require rigorous experimentation and validation. AI can aid in this process by analyzing experimental data and suggesting potential avenues for exploration, but the actual conduct of experiments and the interpretation of their outcomes remain human responsibilities. Researchers must evaluate AI-generated hypotheses and conduct controlled studies to verify their validity, a process that involves meticulous attention to detail and critical thinking.
4. Serendipitous Insights: Many medical discoveries have historically been serendipitous, resulting from unexpected observations and

chance encounters. While AI can enhance systematic data analysis, it cannot replicate the serendipity that sometimes leads to major breakthroughs. The ability to recognize and act on unexpected findings requires a human touch, with researchers often drawing on their experience and intuition to pursue unconventional paths.

5. Ethical and Contextual Considerations: The application of AI in medicine must navigate ethical and contextual considerations that require human judgment. Decisions about patient care, treatment options, and research directions often involve complex ethical dilemmas that AI cannot resolve on its own. Human oversight is essential to ensure that AI-driven insights are applied in ways that are ethically sound and contextually appropriate.
6. Limitations in Current AI Technology: Current AI technologies have limitations that prevent them from solving all medical mysteries. These limitations include difficulties in understanding complex biological systems, integrating heterogeneous data sources, and making sense of incomplete or noisy data. While AI can provide valuable tools for analyzing data, its conclusions must be interpreted and validated by human experts who understand the broader context of medical research.
7. Role of Human Intuition and Experience: Human intuition and experience play critical roles in medical discovery. Experienced researchers and clinicians can draw on their deep knowledge and expertise to make informed decisions, recognize subtle patterns, and generate innovative ideas. AI can augment this process by providing data-driven insights, but it cannot replace the nuanced understanding that comes from years of hands-on experience in the field.
8. Need for Continuous Learning and Adaptation: The medical field is constantly evolving, with new diseases emerging, treatments being developed, and knowledge expanding. AI systems need continuous updates and retraining to stay current with the latest developments. Human researchers and clinicians are essential

for driving this ongoing learning process, ensuring that AI tools remain relevant and effective in addressing new medical challenges.

9. Facilitation Rather than Substitution: Ultimately, AI should be seen as a facilitator of medical discovery rather than a substitute for human ingenuity. It can enhance the capabilities of researchers and clinicians, providing powerful tools for data analysis and hypothesis generation. However, the core of medical discovery remains rooted in human creativity, curiosity, and collaboration.

In summary, while AI has the potential to revolutionize medical research and clinical practice by accelerating data analysis and pattern recognition, it is not a panacea for solving all medical mysteries. Human researchers and clinicians are indispensable for driving innovation, conducting rigorous experiments, and making ethical decisions. AI serves as a valuable tool that enhances human capabilities, but the essence of medical discovery lies in the collaborative efforts and creative insights of the human mind.

REFERENCES AND FURTHER READING

Book References:

1. Deep Learning by Ian Goodfellow, Yoshua Bengio, and Aaron Courville. MIT Press
2. Introduction to Machine Learning with Python: A Guide for Data Scientists, Andreas Muller, O'Reilly
3. Computer Vision: A Modern Approach, Forsyth / Ponce, Pearson
4. Understanding Natural Language Processing (Machine Learning and Deep Learning Perspectives), T V Geetha, Pearson
5. Explainable Artificial Intelligence (XAI): What we know and what is left to attain Trustworthy Artificial Intelligence, Sajid Ali et.al. Information Fusion, Elsevier
6. AI Healthcare Applications and Security, Ethical, and Legal Considerations, Babita Singla, Kumar Shalender, IGI Global
7. Generative and Active Artificial Intelligence: Unveiling Myths and Opportunities, Ana Carla Bliacheriene, Luciano Vieira de Araújo

Website References:

1. History of artificial intelligence.
   https://www.britannica.com/science/history-of-artificial-intelligence

2. What Is The Impact Of Artificial Intelligence On Society?
   https://bernardmarr.com/what-is-the-impact-of-artificial-intelligence-ai-on-society/

3. Drawbacks of Artificial Intelligence and Their Potential Solutions in the Healthcare Sector. Biomedical Materials & Devices https://link.springer.com/article/10.1007/s44174-023-00063-2

4. Deep Blue.
https://www.ibm.com/history/deep-blue

5. What Is Edge AI and How Does It Work?
https://blogs.nvidia.com/blog/what-is-edge-ai/

6. Machine Learning Tutorial.
https://www.geeksforgeeks.org/machine-learning/

7. Introducing Deep Learning and Neural Networks — Deep Learning for Rookies.
https://towardsdatascience.com/

8. Generative AI.
https://www.javatpoint.com/generative-ai

9. Is our healthcare system broken? Harvard Health Publishing.
https://www.health.harvard.edu/blog/is-our-healthcare-system-broken-202107132542

10. AI in healthcare. Foresee medical.
https://www.foreseemed.com/artificial-intelligence-in-healthcare

11. AI Healthcare Startups: Redefining Medical Innovation.
https://adamfard.com/blog/ai-healthcare-startups

12. Explainable Artificial Intelligence (XAI), DARPA.
https://www.darpa.mil/program/explainable-artificial-intelligence

13. Wikimedia Commons.
https://commons.wikimedia.org/

14. Unsplash.
https://unsplash.com

15. Financial News Media.
https://www.globenewswire.com/

16. Edge Delta.
https://edgedelta.com/company/blog/how-much-data-is-created-per-day

17. The Physicians Foundation.
https://physiciansfoundation.org/

18. The World Health Organization.
https://www.who.int/

19. Artificial Intelligence for Healthcare: Insights from India.
https://www.chathamhouse.org/2020/07/artificial-intelligence-healthcare-insights-india/references

20. Gershgorn, D. (2018), 'If AI is going to be the world's doctor, it needs better textbooks', Quartz, 6 September 2018
https://qz.com/1367177/if-ai-is-going-to-be-the-worlds-doctor-it-needsbetter-textbooks

21. Siddiqui, F. R. (2008), 'Denied treatment, Dalit woman dies', The Times of India, 25 April 2008
https://timesofindia.indiatimes.com/city/lucknow/Denied-treatment-Dalit-woman-dies/ articleshow/2980771.cms

22. Hart, D. R. (2017), 'If you're not a white male, artificial intelligence's use in healthcare could be dangerous', Quartz, 10 July 2017
https://qz.com/1023448/if-youre-not-a-white-male-artificialintelligences-use-in-healthcare-could-be-dangerous

INDEX

Clustering, 53–54, 89, 203

www.ingramcontent.com/pod-product-compliance
Ingram Content Group UK Ltd.
Pitfield, Milton Keynes, MK11 3LW, UK
UKHW060117010826
14089UKWH00004B/36

9 798897 248667